REAL EXERCISE FOR REAL PEOPLE

HOW TO ORDER
Single copies may be ordered from Prima Publishing, P.O. Box 1260BK, Rocklin, CA 95677; telephone (916) 632-4400. Quantity discounts are also available. On your letterhead, include information concerning the intended use of the books and the number of books you wish to purchase.

REAL EXERCISE FOR REAL PEOPLE

Finding Your Optimum Level of Physical Activity for a Lifetime of Healthy Living

Peter Francis, Ph.D.
Lorna Francis, Ph.D.

PRIMA PUBLISHING

To Cameron and Ashley, who have taught us
more about ourselves and about life in the
few short years they have been around than
we ever learned in the many years before.

Origianlly published by Prima Publishing in 1988 under the title *If It Hurts Don't Do It.*

PRIMA PUBLISHING and colophon are trademarks of Prima Communications, Inc.

Library of Congress Cataloging-in-Publication Data

Francis, Peter R.
   Real exercise for real people: finding your optimum level of physical fitness for a lifetime of healthy living / Peter Francis and Lorna Francis.
     p.   cm.
   ISBN 0-7615-0331-5
   1. Exercise. 2. Physical Fitness. I. Francis, Lorna. II. Title.
GV481.F695   1996
613.7'1—dc20   96-613
                                               CIP

96 97 98 99 00 01 AA 10 9 8 7 6 5 4 3 2 1
Printed in the United States of America

CONTENTS

Chapter 1
GAIN WITHOUT PAIN   1

Did you know that

- *40 percent of the American adult population doesn't exercise at all?*

- *another 40 percent exercises sporadically*

- *40–50 percent of those who join formal exercise programs drop out within 6 months to a year*

- *the majority of fitness enthusiasts have the mistaken belief that exercise has to hurt to be doing any goods*

Why do so many people choose not to exercise knowing it could make them look and feel better, even add years to their lives? What led to the belief that exercise has to hurt in order to be beneficial? These questions are carefully explored in this chapter. We then introduce our unique four-step approach to life-time fitness.

Chapter 2
SETTING YOUR EXERCISE GOALS   11

Have you written out your exercise goals? Are they Specific? Measurable? Action-oriented? Realistic? Timed? If you're searching for a way to stick with your exercise program, you'll want to learn the SMART System for setting exercise goals.

Chapter 3
TESTING YOUR PHYSICAL LIMITATIONS   21

Lying on your back, can you lift one leg up to the ceiling until it is vertical without bending either knee? If you can't, it may be one of the reasons your lower back bothers you occasionally.

Can you reach behind your head with your right arm and touch your left shoulder blade with your fingertips? If you can't and you play tennis, you may be a candidate for tennis elbow, or if you swim the front crawl, you may find yourself getting very tired very quickly.

We take you through an interesting series of tests designed to evaluate your readiness to exercise. You'll be able to examine your health history, posture, the tightness and strength of certain muscles as well as your aerobic fitness level. Specific exercises are then recommended for any deficiency you might have.

How do you decide which exercises to do? If you're like most people, you select exercises everyone else is doing even though you're not quite sure why you're doing them. To avoid boredom, injury, and disillusionment with exercise, you must make discriminate choices about your exercises, physical activities, and even your exercise equipment. We discuss the fact that each and every exercise should be done for a specific purpose and we offer guidelines for making discriminate choices.

Do you neglect to stretch before participating in vigorous physical activity? Do you bounce when you stretch? Do you do standing toe touches? If you answered "yes" to any of these questions, read this chapter. We discuss the benefits of stretching as well as the adverse effects of failing to stretch. We guide you through the dos and don'ts of specific stretching exercises and we draw your attention to the ten most unwanted stretches in your exercise program.

Sit-ups reduce the amount of fat around your stomach. True or false?
"Going for the burn" (working a muscle until it burns) will make your muscles stronger. True or false?
Women who lift weights will develop large bulging muscles. True or false?
If you answered "true" to any of these statements, this chapter is for you. We clear up a number of exercise myths and discuss dos and

*don'ts of muscle toning. We introduce you to appropriate strength
exercises and to some of the most undesirable exercise positions.*

*Do you find yourself hurting every time you start a new exercise pro-
grams? While your heart and muscles adjust fairly readily to the new
stresses of vigorous activity, your bones, tendons, ligaments, and
joints take considerably longer. We introduce the idea of a pre-aerobic
program which is designed to adequately prepare your body for vigorous physical activities.*

*How long, how often, and how hard should you exercise aerobically?
The answers are not quite as simple as you might think. We teach
you how to maximize aerobic benefits while at the same time mini-
mizing the risk of injury. We then introduce various physical activities and discuss their advantages and potential risks. This
information will help you become a discriminating exerciser.*

*Losing weight seems to be the number one goal of the majority
of people who take part in exercise programs. We've devoted an
entire chapter to this concern. You will learn what exercise can
do for your weight.*

*Sticking with an exercise program can be difficult. We share a num-
ber of strategies that will help you stay with your program.
For example, if you like to walk or jog, you can do any of the
following activities to give your exercise a little lift.*

- *take a friend along*
- *listen to music or motivational/self-improvement audiotapes*
- *if you're improving certain skills such as your vocabulary or accounting skills, create small cue cards that fit in your pocket or in the palm of your hand and test your memory while you exercise*
- *use the time for brainstorming new ideas for your work, home, family, or yourself*

FOREWORD

Congratulations, you have just acquired a book by two of the most credible and trustworthy names in the industry of health and fitness.

Fitness is a lifestyle which enhances overall health. There are hundreds of health and fitness books, videos, and television programs on the market and it can be confusing to know which program is correct for you. This makes it difficult to select the appropriate workout or product that will answer your questions and help you reach your personal fitness goals.

Everyone has questions and concerns about their own health and fitness goals. I like to get my aerobic exercise by crosstraining the stepper with the treadmill, whereas my friend enjoys walking on the beach. You need to remember that you are unique and it is important to develop a fitness program that is adaptable to your lifestyle.

Real Exercise for Real People allows you to be unique and create your own fitness program to fit your lifestyle. Whether you're a beginning or advanced exerciser, you will find the resources and information in this book to help you build a safe, effective program.

Drs. Peter and Lorna Francis have been dedicated to the scientific study of fitness. In fact, most of the principles for safe exercise that we have today come from their scientific study of this field. Because these programs are backed up by many years of invaluable laboratory research, they will help you reach your fitness goals by becoming a part of your everyday life!

Drs. Peter and Lorna Francis are to fitness what the Good Housekeeping Seal is to products.

Tamilee Webb, M.A.
Ms. Buns of Steel

ACKNOWLEDGMENTS

Many people have helped us to complete the work that has culminated with the publication of this book. Each of us was profoundly affected by our parents. Dorothy Stewart and Alfred Francis are no longer with us, but we learned a great deal about love, loyalty, and bravery from the two of them. Caroline Francis and Gordon Stewart continue to share their gifts of perseverance and determination with us. All four of our parents encouraged us to be the best we could be in whatever we might choose to do with our lives.

The two of us have been fortunate to have been associated with the faculties of three fine universities: Iowa State University, the University of Oregon, and San Diego State University. We learned much from our talented colleagues, and even more from the thousands of students who have challenged us with their unquenchable thirst for knowledge.

A special thanks to Michael Buono, Ph.D., for his valuable review of the physiological information in this book, and to Bobbe Sommer, Ph.D., for sharing her expertise in the area of goal setting. Peter is also indebted to the Sports Science Division of the United States Olympic Committee, which, under the outstanding leadership of Charles Dillman, Ph.D., has provided funding for the research involving elite athletes that has been conducted in the Biomechanics Laboratory at San Diego State University.

The following individuals have also made significant contributions to this book: Ben Dominitz, President of Prima Publishing, and his colleagues have shown remarkable insight into the underlying concepts covered in our writings, and they have been enormously helpful with all the chores of editing; Mary Fischer, an aspiring young writer who helped us get this project off the ground; and Uniak for its wonderful photography.

A special thanks to our physically fit models, Dee, Diane, Carl and Stan. Diane is an accomplished aerobics instructor, and Stan is one of our graduate students as well as a gifted athlete. Professor Emeritus Carl Benton and his wife Dee, who have been retired for some time, serve as fine examples of the health benefits of many years of continuous physical activity.

We would also like to offer our thanks to Pari and Amir, who provide our two children with endless love and attention during the time we spend teaching and writing. Finally, we cannot miss the opportunity to thank our children, Cameron and Ashley. We hope that some of the wisdom they have brought us has found its way into the pages of this book.

A Special Acknowledgment

The authors would like to offer their most sincere thanks for all the encouragement and support they have received over the past five years from Reebok International. In 1983, we had the good fortune to meet Angel Martinez, who was an executive of a then fledgling sports shoe company. At that time he told us about the long-term goals of the company under the direction of its remarkable president, Paul Fireman. We discovered that we all had a common goal of improving public education in the safety aspects of sport and physical fitness. Mr. Fireman agreed to provide financial support for a research project that was designed to examine possible causes of injuries in aerobic dance programs. When this was successfully completed, Reebok offered to continue its support for our research, and we have carried out a variety of investigations involving aerobic dance, step training, slide training, racewalking, tennis, and volleyball. The Reebok organization has also provided opportunities for us to travel throughout the world to present the results of research conducted by us and other exercise scientists.

All too often Big Business has a reputation for becoming dehumanized during periods of expansion. Reebok started with little more than a tradition of craftsmanship that began at the beginning of the century in England, but under the leadership of Paul Fireman it has become one of the best-known business success stories of recent times. In spite of this phenomenal growth, the company has steadfastly maintained its commitment to its goal of supporting research and education. As a result of the resources that Reebok has made available, a number of our graduate students have received financial support that has helped them with the expenses of their education. Reebok has also given us the opportunity to pursue some of our own educational goals, and most recently has given considerable help with the photography for this book. Our professional relationship with Reebok International has been a gratifying confirmation of our belief that "Good guys can finish first!" Thank you for everything.

Chapter 1

GAIN WITHOUT PAIN

"I know that exercise is important, and I have been meaning to try an exercise program, but I just haven't found the time to start one yet."—L. S., Iowa

"I have tried a number of exercise programs, but I haven't found one that didn't become boring after a few weeks." — V. M., Illinois

"Are you joking! Can you imagine me in one of those spandex outfits!"—J. N., New Jersey

"I love to exercise and I never miss a day, even though I suffer from constant pain in my shins."—S. B., California

Don't be fooled by the media hype about the "fitness boom." We recently asked a number of people of all ages about their exercise habits, and the comments above are typical. In spite of the endless procession on television and in magazines of people becoming healthier and more attractive as the result of daily exercise, don't feel left out if you don't seem to be one of them. And don't think it's unusual if you haven't been satisfied with the results of your exercise programs.

1

Did you know that:

- 40 percent of the American adult population doesn't exercise at all?

- another 40 percent exercises sporadically?

- 40 to 50 percent of those people who join formal exercise programs drop out within six months to a year?

- the majority of people have the mistaken belief that exercise has to hurt in order to be doing any good?

Why do so many people avoid exercise, even though they seem to believe it could make them look and feel better, even add years to their lives? Why do so many others find it impossible to stick with exercise programs? Why do so many people think that exercise has to hurt? After researching these questions for years, we have come to the conclusion that exercise is one of the most misunderstood concepts in our society.

Why do these misconceptions surround exercise? Surely, there is no shortage of information. The shelves in the fitness sections of libraries, bookstores, and video stores are full. Television shows and newspapers regularly feature fitness topics, and dozens of magazines are published especially for the exercise enthusiast. Scientific research is constantly providing new information about the benefits of exercise, and it seems as if every week another movie or TV star has found the secret to health, fitness, and beauty. But if you have tried valiantly to keep up with this deluge of information, you will have noticed that a great deal of what is being said seems to be contradictory.

We believe the real problem is that too much information is available right now and the average person doesn't have sufficient knowledge to distinguish fact from popular fantasy. Of course, most reasonably intelligent people are leery of an "unrepeatable offer" that concludes with "Yes—I enclose my check for $29.95. Rush me your secret formula for lifelong fitness, beauty, and success." But we're continually bombarded with word of "discoveries," "inventions," and "secrets" that sound convincing, even though they're often either deliberately misleading or simply unsubstantiated by any reputable expert in the field of health and fitness.

In our roles as members of the physical education faculty at a large university, we are continually struck by the fact that many bright young students have completely unrealistic expectations about what exercise can do for them. It is hardly surprising that millions of others who are out of touch with the sciences are equally naive about something that can have such a profound effect on their health and well-being. The major purpose of this book is to dispel many of the popular myths about exercise. We believe that sensible exercise is a way for each of us to take greater control over our personal health and enrich the quality of our lives.

A New Approach

As a result of our ongoing work in the area of fitness, we believe that you can maintain lifelong physical fitness through a new and exciting program of thoroughly enjoyable, pain-free exercise. Our approach is based not on special gimmicks, nor on the "secrets" of Hollywood gurus or mysterious clinics tucked away in remote corners of Europe, but on sound science and common sense. Our program represents the culmination of many years of research by us and many other credible experts all over the world. Our goal has been to make the most up-to-date scientific information as understandable as possible. In recent years, we have had the pleasure of working with people of all ages and all fitness levels, from senior citizens to Olympic champions. This exciting new approach has helped them and it can help you.

Our approach is based on the simple fact that the most important step in understanding what exercise can and can't do for you is to better understand your own unique body. Each one of us should be concerned about our own body, which is different from any other body on this planet. It differs in size and shape from any other. It is equipped to do some things better than other bodies, and it may have imperfections that prevent it from performing some activities as well as the bodies of exceptionally gifted individuals. In just the same way that you have your own special preferences in food and music, your body will tend to dictate the types of exercise that it likes. As you know only too well, your body has its own unmistakable way of letting you know when you are trying to force it to perform in ways it simply can't handle.

After you have learned more about the make-up of your own unique body, we will help you design a personalized exercise program that is exactly right for you. This will allow you to prescribe exercises for your unique body in much the same way that a doctor prescribes medication for the unique symptoms of each patient. Most exercise books, tapes, and videos available at this time provide exercise routines that are supposedly suitable for anyone who chooses to use them. We believe that this is equivalent to a doctor prescribing aspirin for every single patient who seeks medical advice. Of course, aspirin is an appropriate treatment for a number of medical problems, but some conditions can be worsened by the indiscriminate use of this common drug. In the same way, many popular exercises are appropriate for most people, but some of the exercises included in many fixed programs can be painful or injurious to individuals who may be anatomically vulnerable.

Another unique aspect of our approach is that you will be able to decide exactly what you want to get out of your own program. We will give you choices so that you can select precisely the best, painfree, enjoyable activities that will help you reach your exercise goals. We will show you what it takes to stick with your program and how you can measure the improvements in fitness that your personalized program will produce.

New Beginning

More than 50 years ago, a number of remarkable individuals in the United States began to advocate the value of physical fitness as the key to good health and well-being. The exploits of pioneers such as Jack LaLane are now the stuff of legends. (Jack recently turned 80, but he still retains his vigor and evangelical zeal for spreading his gospel of physical fitness). The early advocates focused mainly on strength and muscular endurance, which at that time had much greater appeal to males than to females. It was not until 30 years later that fitness emerged as an important issue for men and women alike.

Why haven't people taken this approach before? Quite simply, it is an idea whose time has come. Scientists have learned more about exercise in the last two or three decades than at any other time in history. We have become increasingly aware of the importance of exercise in our sedentary society, especially as it relates to the health of our hearts and lungs.

Aerobic exercise was a concept introduced in the '70s that set the entire health movement in motion. Dr. Kenneth Cooper launched the idea into the mainstream with his series of best-selling books on aerobics, as did the late Jim Fixx with *The Complete Book of Running*. Running sparked exercise consciousness on a grand scale. The idea of prolonged exercise intended to stimulate the heart and lungs emerged from near obscurity to catch the imagination of the public. The sedentary lifestyle of most people, their imprudent diets, and increasing levels of stress had made heart disease a major killer in America. The yearly number of deaths from heart disease in this country was 50 percent greater than the combined American death toll in World War I, World War II, and the Korean and Vietnamese conflicts. Suddenly, aerobic exercise was a way for people to regain some control of their physical destinies and create visible changes in their bodies. Millions of Americans took to the streets and running tracks as the jogging craze spearheaded the growing fitness boom. The words *distance* and *pace* became new topics of conversation and new criteria by which to impress friends.

Aerobic dance followed running in popularity and today attracts an estimated 20 million Americans, most of them women. This vibrant, exciting form of exercise was introduced in 1969 by Jacki Sorensen, who choreographed exercise routines to music. It was Sorensen who coined the phrase "aerobic dance," while Jane Fonda popularized the idea of working out to music with her best-selling videotapes and books. Millions of aerobic dancers poured into clubs and spas to be a part of this multi-billion-dollar industry that offered fitness, fun, and fashion.

The popularity of running and aerobic dance revived interest in other fitness activities such as weight training, bicycling, swimming, and walking. More recently, newer forms of exercise such as step training and slide training have expanded the options of people who prefer to exercise to music. The big jump in sales of exercise equipment is evidence of this trend. State-of-the-art technology has led to sophisticated features on rowing machines, treadmills, and bikes that keep track of the distance you have covered, your pulse rate, and the number of calories you have burned. Some offer words of encouragement; others have color television sets to entertain you while you exercise. Even swimmers can enjoy their favorite music with waterproof radios. Not only have sales of exercise equipment skyrocketed, but sports footwear and clothing have become the vanguard of the fashion industry.

Some of us remember the late '70s and early '80s as the "aerobic Camelot" when we ran, danced, swam, and cycled farther and faster pursuing health, happiness, and dreams of eternal youth. We rediscovered ancient and mystic wizards ensconced in murky gyms that were remnants of a former fitness epoch. We found dazzling enchantresses who stepped to earth from the silver screen to teach us wondrous things that even to this day are beyond the comprehension of mortal men and women of science. It seemed as if it would never end. But it did!

In scholarly articles in medical journals and lectures at professional conferences, doctors and researchers were reporting that many exercise enthusiasts were getting hurt. In fact, orthopedic surgeons attributed a dramatic increase in patient load to the jogging craze, and one claimed that the injury toll resulting from a celebrity's exercise video tapes was "putting his kids through college." In some activities, as many as 70 percent of participants had apparently been injured. Why? One of the characteristics of the fitness boom of the '70s was a peculiar "Rambo mentality" in all areas of fitness. The notion of "No pain, no gain" caught on and remains the prevailing, though uninformed, attitude toward exercise. The media blitz surrounding exercise was in part responsible for this warrior attitude. Adding fuel to the fire were a number of larger-than-life professional sports personalities and quasi-military screen characters whose contempt for pain was somehow an integral element of their apparent physical fitness. As health club instructors chanted the exhortation "Go for the burn!" more and more people became convinced that pain was the price that Nature extracted in return for the gift of fitness. Indeed, for a masochistic few, "purification through pain" had assumed a kind of mystic significance in their quest for self-improvement.

Another unfortunate effect of the Rambo mentality was an emerging belief that if some exercise is good, a lot more must be better. Many enthusiasts seemed to accept that if strong muscles were good, bigger and stronger muscles were better. The resounding crashes of pumping iron shook the sweat-soaked gyms. If 5 miles of running was good for you, then 10 or 20 miles was better. Hundreds of thousands flocked to run marathons. If a couple of aerobic dance sessions each week was good, six or seven classes a week was better. Clubs and spas pulsed with the electrified beat of popular music. Unfortunately, in their haste to follow the crowd, many people forgot to ask why they were doing these things, and they rarely took the trouble to ask how they should be doing them.

Much to the surprise of many people who thought that jogging was the way for everyone to become physically fit, the craze began to subside. In fact, running experienced a sharp downward trend in 1984, the year Jim Fixx collapsed on a Vermont road and died of a heart attack. Many joggers became disillusioned, wondering whether this kind of exercise lived up to its hype. They were not really seeing and feeling the benefits promised by the running gurus. Instead, they were experiencing aches and pains and had become just plain bored with their exercise programs. For many, the novelty of exercise had worn off. Something was gravely wrong when a whole new area of medical specialization, sports medicine, owed much of its popularity to the casualties of this well-meaning but misdirected movement. And when a flock of injury suits against health clubs and fitness spas were finding their way into the courts, an alternative demanded to be heard.

The Four-Step Approach to Life-long Fitness

For almost 20 years, we have been involved in research in the areas of exercise and sport. During that time, we have lectured to audiences around the world and have met many thousands of exercise enthusiasts who are quite knowledgeable about some of the scientific principles of fitness. Most people know, for example, that aerobic activities are good for the heart. Many accept that stretching and strengthening are also important to total fitness—although not everyone actually incorporates these into his or her program. Few people seem to understand the full fitness picture, however. We have found that many people don't understand the limitations of various physical activities or the exact purpose for many specific exercises.

Quite simply, four key elements are necessary for establishing an effective, lifetime exercise program. They are:

1. Realistic, personal goal setting.

2. Personalized fitness assessment.

3. Discriminate exercise and physical activity.

4. Self-motivation.

In order to devise your own effective and safe exercise program, you must select exercise and physical activities based on the results of fitness tests and your unique exercise goals. And of course you need workable strategies that will keep you going from day to day. Before you start any exercise program, you should ask yourself these four very important questions:

1. What are my exercise goals? (goal setting)

2. Is my body ready to achieve my exercise goals? (self-testing)

3. Exactly what must I do to accomplish my exercise goals? discriminate exercise and physical activity)

4. What can I do to stick with my exercise goals? (self-motivation)

What will our program do for you?

First, we will help you increase your commitment to making regular exercise a part of your life. Without commitment, maintaining an exercise program is very difficult. We will help you set realistic exercise goals. People who set unrealistic goals are inevitably disappointed. We will also help you follow through on your goals.

Second, we will teach you how to examine the most important exercise equipment you own: your body. We will help you determine whether your body is ready for regular, vigorous exercise. Many exercise enthusiasts, including well-trained athletes, experience injuries because of slight alignment problems that in many cases can be detected with a few simple tests. Why not begin your exercise program with a finely tuned instrument and reduce your risk of injury?

Third, we will provide you with safe, comfortable, and carefully chosen exercises that will help fine-tune your body so that you can improve both your health and the quality of your life. Contrary to popular belief, physical fitness is not a single component of your health; it is actually made up of three separate factors: flexibility, strength, and aerobic fitness. We will help you increase your overall fitness by improving each one of these separate components. In Chapter 5 we will discuss specific ways that you can improve your flexibility, and in Chapter 6 we will introduce you to specific exercises for improving your strength. In Chapter 8 we will show you how to improve your aerobic fitness using enjoyable, pain-free activities that you can select on the basis of your exercise goals, your special interests, and your own unique body.

Fourth, we will provide you with techniques that will motivate you to stick with your program. We will introduce you to strategies that will help you look forward to your exercise each day. This will ensure that you can go on reaping the benefits of your personalized exercise program for the rest of what we hope will be a full, healthy, and happy lifetime.

Chapter 2

SETTING YOUR EXERCISE GOALS

Have you noticed that many people seem to have rather vague ideas about what they would like to accomplish in their lives? For example, many people would like to be "rich," "successful," or "happy," but they often have difficulty defining exactly what they mean by riches, success, and happiness. When we questioned various people about their exercise goals, they tended to be equally vague. Many told us that they wanted to be "healthy" and "fit," but when we asked a dozen people to define health and fitness, we got 12 entirely different answers!

Have you also noticed that many of the same people who have trouble telling you exactly what they hope to achieve in life are the same people who lament the fact that their dreams never seem to come true? We have found that many of the people who tell us they have never succeeded in reaching their exercise goals also have the most trouble telling us how they planned to reach them. This common state of affairs can be illustrated by the results of studies of both successful and unsuccessful individuals in many different fields. Research has shown that people who clearly know what they want and how they are going to get it are most likely to achieve their goals. For this reason it is important to decide exactly what you want in life. This is known as goal setting.

11

SMART Goals

In order to develop a lifetime commitment to exercise, you must set exercise goals. A number of different strategies can help you do this, but we have a favorite technique that is often recommended by experts in the field of self-improvement. The "Smart System" is based on the concept that achievable goals should be:

Specific
Measurable
Action-oriented
Realistic
Timed

Specific Goals

Goals must be specific in order to be achievable. We have often heard people say that they wanted "to get in shape." In shape for what? For competitive skiing, to fit into a new bikini, or to play touch football on the weekend without getting out of breath? People have also told us that they wanted to improve their health. What aspect of their health? Do they want to reduce stress, lessen the risk of heart disease, or get rid of low back pain? Unless you clearly define your goals by specifying exactly what you want to gain from your exercise program, you will have trouble deciding on the best means of achieving those goals.

Measurable Goals

Your goals must be measurable; otherwise, you have no way of judging your progress toward achieving them. Fortunately, most carefully defined exercise goals are measurable. For example, you can measure weight loss with your bathroom scale. If you wanted to be even more precise, you could have an expert estimate the amount of fat you have lost using skinfold callipers or a technique that involves weighing you while you are suspended underwater. If you wish to measure the changes in the girth of your abdomen or your thighs, you can do so with a tape measure. You can even use the change in the fit of your clothes as a form of girth measurement. In this book we will provide you with ways of measuring improvements in other aspects of your physical fitness.

Action-Oriented Goals

Actions speak louder than words! This old adage was never more true than when it is applied to exercise. Wishes and dreams are not enough. You must have a plan of action that you can follow as you strive to meet your own unique goals. Studies of successful individuals have shown that the most effective way to prepare an action plan is to write it down. As a first step, write down your "General Action Plan," which will determine the type of program best suited for your goals. For example, if you want to be more supple, you need to begin a stretching program or maybe a yoga program. If you want to look like Mr. Universe, you need to get started on a weight training program. Once you have selected the type of program, list all the possible ways to accomplish your action plan. Are you going to join a class or a club? Read a book or watch a home video? Enlist the help of a personal trainer?

When you have completed your General Action Plan, the next step is to write out "Weekly Action Plans." We have included pages that can be photocopied for this purpose in the Exercise Goals at the back of this book; an excellent selection of personal planning calendars is also available in stationery stores. These ringbinders usually include pages that can be used for action plans for any kind of goal setting—business, personal affairs, or exercise.

If you have not exercised for some time, a typical Weekly Action Plan might indicate your intention to walk for 10 to 15 minutes on Monday, Wednesday, and Friday with your neighbor. Perhaps you will also plan to spend less time watching television and work daily on those exercises that have been recommended by your doctor for your low back pain. If you are already in excellent condition, your weekly action plan might include a one-mile swim on Monday and Wednesday, a five-mile jog on Tuesday, a ten-mile bike ride on Thursday, one hour of weight training on

Friday, a leisurely walk with your nearest and dearest at the local scenic spot on Saturday, and a well-earned rest on Sunday.

Review your action plan at the end of each week. Did you accomplish what you wanted? If you did, you'll have the satisfaction of knowing that you're making progress toward your exercise goals. What if you were unable to achieve what you wanted? Don't become discouraged. Researchers have found that it takes at least six to eight weeks for us to change an old behavior pattern. Try to stick to your action plan for at least two months before throwing in the towel. Above all, if things aren't going well after a couple of months, don't assume that exercise can't work for you. Go back and review your General Action Plan. Is it still what you want to accomplish? Check your Weekly Action Plans. Have you made unreasonable demands on yourself? You've got to find out what is right for you, so don't be afraid to make changes along the way if something just isn't working.

Realistic Goals

Your goals must be realistic if you expect to achieve them. Each of us exercises for various reasons. Some of us want to be thinner, stronger, or shapelier. Others want to reduce low back pain, psychological stress, or the risk of heart disease. Still others enjoy the social opportunities offered by some activities. Of course, you can exercise with more than one purpose in mind, but the key to realistic goal setting is understanding what exercise can and can't do for you.

Predictably, many of the people who have quit exercise programs appear to have been disillusioned with exercise because it didn't give them the results they expected. In most cases either the exercise goals they had set or the means they had used to reach their goals were totally unrealistic.

Take Victor, for instance. He was a military reservist who was due to go to camp in three weeks. He joined Lorna's conditioning class hoping to lose thirty pounds before going to camp. Victor was extremely disappointed to learn that he would have to exercise vigorously and continuously for almost every hour that he was awake for the entire three weeks to lose thirty pounds of fat. Unfortunately, in his present condition, Victor would have either collapsed from exhaustion or hurt himself long before losing a fraction of the weight.

Julie was another memorable example of someone with unrealistic goals. She was generally slim, but she had unusually broad hips. It was apparent that she was not overweight but she was obviously born with a stocky frame. She came to one of our workshops and told us that she had been attending two aerobic dance classes every day in the hope of slimming down to a trimmer figure. She was extremely discouraged with her lack of progress and she wanted to know what she was doing wrong. Julie didn't understand that although exercise can do many things, it can't change a person's basic genetic makeup. Someone who is born pear-shaped is destined to be pear-shaped for life. Through diet and exercise you can change the size of the pear (from large to small), but you can't change the shape of the pear! The glamorous personalities who adorn the covers of popular magazines and exercise books inherited their unique body shapes from their parents. With conscientious exercise they are able, like the rest of us, to maintain their bodies in the best condition possible within the constraints of their basic body shapes. We must all be realistic about what exercise can and can't do for us.

Not only your goals but the way you plan to achieve them must be realistic. One of the most common myths in our society is that we can selectively "spot reduce" fat in certain areas of the body by doing specific exercises. For many people, weight loss is a realistic goal, but it is completely unrealistic to expect to be able to selectively lose weight around the abdomen through endless sessions of sit-ups and side bends. You simply can't pick and choose the spots where you would like to lose fat. We'll discuss spot reducing further in Chapter 6.

Our good friend Frank chose an unrealistic way of achieving his goal of losing thirty or forty pounds. At the height of the jogging craze, his buddies in the office convinced him that running was the best way for anyone to lose weight quickly. Assured that he could look like his lean and healthy running companions, he began running several miles every day. He bore the predictable pain and suffered a knee injury long before shedding a single pound of fat. Now Frank is more careful with his diet. He walks to the office every other day, cycles every weekend, and has never looked or felt better during his whole adult life.

Timed Goals

Finally, if you develop specific, measurable, action-oriented, realistic exercise goals, you will inevitably develop a great deal of confidence in the outcome of your efforts. As a final challenge, you can demonstrate your new-found confidence and genuine commitment to your program by setting a target date for achieving your goals. Select a specific day, month, and year. Write it down!

Some years ago Olga asked us to assist her in designing a personalized exercise program that would help her with her favorite sport, cycling. At that time one of her goals was to enter the 75-mile race from Tecate to Ensenada, Mexico, and to finish in five hours. Much to her delight, her actual time was 15 minutes better than she had anticipated. She is continuing to train hard and has rarely missed training sessions through injury or lack of interest. The most striking aspect of this story is that Olga was not particularly well-organized or determined when we first met her. Now she believes that her successful exercise program has taught her valuable lessons that are having an extremely positive effect on other aspects of her personal and professional life.

How Can the SMART System Work for You?

Let's look at an example of how SMART goal setting works. Suppose your goal is to lose weight. Is that a specific goal? Yes, but it could be more specific. Presumably you want to lose fat rather than muscle. How much do you want to lose? Let's say you want to lose ten pounds. Now you have a specific goal. Is your goal measurable? Yes, but how are you going to measure you weight loss? Even though you may be most interested in the amount of fat you will lose rather than the total number of pounds, you may still decide that your bathroom scale is the easiest way to keep track of your progress. Now your goal is measurable. Is your goal action-oriented? It is if you have a strategy for losing the weight. If you reduce your daily food intake by 500 calories and take a gentle walk every day, you can expect to lose between one to two pounds of fat each week. Is your goal of losing ten pounds of fat a realistic goal? Yes it is, provided you give yourself adequate time to lose it. In fact, you can expect that it will take as much as two and a half months to lose the ten pounds. In Chapter 9, we will give you more specific information about the relationship between the amount of fat you lose and the resulting change in your weight, as measured by your bathroom scale. This brings us to the final step of goal setting: timing your goal. State the day, month, and year you plan to achieve that goal. Now, that wasn't so hard was it?

Getting Started

Step 1: Select your own specific exercise goal or goals. Different people have many and varied exercise goals. Here are some that people have told us about:

- weight control
- improved appearance
- improved strength and muscle tone
- improved flexibility
- improved cardiovascular fitness
- improved sports performance
- stress reduction
- improved self-esteem
- quitting smoking
- overcoming alcohol and substance abuse

You may have other goals that are important to you, and many people have more than one exercise goal.

Step 2: How are you going to measure your accomplishments? Each of the goals in the preceding list is measurable. We will discuss measuring techniques more specifically in Chapters 3, 8, and 9.

Step 3: What is your action plan? You will have to decide on the appropriate program to accomplish your goal. Are you going to begin a stretching, strength, or aerobic program? Are you going to do it on your own, with a neighbor, while watching a TV program or video, or are you going to join a health club? How many times a week are you going to exercise? For how long will you exercise, and how hard are you going to work? The answers will all become clearer as you continue to read this book.

Step 4: Is your goal realistic? Again, you will be able to answer this question more accurately when you have finished this book. Remember, not only does your goal have to be realistic but so does the method you use for accomplishing it. Selecting discriminate exercises and physical activities is a must!

Step 5: Time your goal. Be realistic about how long it will take you to accomplish your goal and set a day, month, and year.

Before reading any further, write out your present exercise goals in the spaces provided below. Follow the five step approach we've just described. Don't worry if you don't know all the answers yet. Do your best, using whatever information you have available to you right now.

1. Your specific exercise goal or goals

2. How will you measure these goals?

3. What's your action plan?
    (a) General Action Plan

(b) Typical Weekly Action Plan

4. Are you convinced that this action plan is realistic? Why?

5. Date for achieving goals

We have provided additional tables like this one in the Exercise Diary in Appendix G so that you can re-evaluate your program at various times in the future. When you have finished reading the book, come back to this chapter and re-examine your present comments in light of what you have learned. If you make some changes on the basis of the information in the following chapters, we will have been successful in getting our message across. Read on and explore the exciting prospects of designing your own personalized program. We hope that your successful participation will give you as much satisfaction as we've had in preparing this practical new approach to exercise.

FIT TIPS

1. The first step to a successful, lifetime commitment to exercise is setting exercise goals.
2. Develop SMART goals: specific, measurable, action-oriented, realistic, and timed.
3. Write your goals on paper, re-evaluate them periodically, and revise them as needed.

Chapter 3

TESTING YOUR PHYSICAL LIMITATIONS

Jeff bought a new ten-speed and set off on a touring holiday of the Oregon coast. After the first two days he had constant pain in his right knee, and on the fifth day he developed a severe pain in his left Achilles tendon. Miserably, he struggled through to the end of the ten-day ordeal. After a couple of weeks of inactivity, Jeff began to ride every day in spite of worsening pain in his knee and heel cord. Eventually he sought medical advice and was fortunately referred to a podiatrist who is also a cycling enthusiast. A careful evaluation indicated that Jeff is severely flat-footed and is rather bowlegged. These conditions can increase a cyclist's vulnerability to the kinds of injuries that Jeff had suffered. His podiatrist prescribed unobtrusive, custom-made arch supports that Jeff now wears inside his shoes, and he showed him how to adjust the cleats on his cycling shoes. He has since enjoyed many months of pain-free cycling.

Jeff was injured *before* he found out that his unique anatomy would inevitably predispose him to injuries the moment he started to pedal a bicycle. Wouldn't it be much easier to find out ahead of time whether you have any anatomical characteristics that make injury likely if you try to do specific activities? The good news is that there are ways of doing just that!

Years of clinical observation have shown that people who do not have proper body alignment are more likely to get hurt during vigorous physical activities than people who do. Jeff the cyclist was a typical example; he could have aptly been considered "an accident waiting to happen." How can you find out whether you have any structural deficiencies?

The most effective way is to seek the assistance of an expert who is experienced in this area. Many medical and paramedical specialists such as orthopedic and osteopathic surgeons, podiatrists, physical therapists, and athletic trainers take a keen interest in the field of exercise and sports fitness. A growing number of these experts are beginning to recognize the need for this kind of evaluation, and many are highly skilled at administering appropriate tests.

Typically, a detailed evaluation would consist of a questionnaire and a series of tests designed to reveal any undesirable characteristics of your muscles, bones, joints, heart, and lungs, and other important physical components of your body. In a clinical setting many of these tests can be made with a high degree of accuracy. Of course, most people will find the expense of such an evaluation difficult to justify. Therefore, we have put together a series of do-it-yourself tests that you can use to carry out your own preliminary evaluation.

The self-testing program consists of a health history questionnaire, a postural analysis, muscle tightness tests, muscle strength tests, and a test for your aerobic fitness level. Don't forget that any evaluation carried out by an untrained individual will invariably miss some problems and incorrectly identify minor things as being problematic. However, many of the tests that we will discuss are modifications of tests that medical professionals use routinely. In their simplified forms, these do-it-yourself tests lack the precision that can be obtained by skilled professionals using clinical instruments, but they do provide extremely useful information about your present level of physical fitness.

Health History Questionnaire

Other sensible remedies will greatly reduce the likelihood of complications arising from many other health problems. The health history questionnaire lists those factors that can lead to complications. If you have any of the problems listed in the questionnaire, it does not mean that you can't exercise, it simply means that a doctor who is familiar with your health history may be able to advise what you should and shouldn't do.

Before engaging in any form of vigorous exercise, you should answer the following questions.

1. Do you have a history of any of the following?

Heart problems?	yes	no
High blood pressure?	yes	no
High blood cholesterol?	yes	no
Respiratory problems?	yes	no
Diabetes?	yes	no
Recent surgery (in the last 3 months)?	yes	no
Major illness or injury (in the last 3 months)?	yes	no
Hospitalization (in the last 3 months)?	yes	no
Any unusual pain or discomfort in the joints?	yes	no

2. Are you over 45 years old (if you are a man); or over 55 years old (if you are a woman)?   yes   no

3. Are you on any prescribed medication that could adversely affect your health while exercising? (If you're unsure, check with your doctor.)   yes   no

4. Are you pregnant?   yes   no

If you answered yes to any of these questions, you are advised to seek medical approval before you participate in any vigorous exercise program. Don't be too concerned about possible consequences at this stage, however. Recent medical research tends to suggest that the benefits of moderate exercise outweigh the risks for the vast majority of people, and so many doctors will encourage you to go ahead with your exercise program. It is likely that your doctor will simply advise some restrictions on certain types of exercise, depending on the nature and severity of your specific problem.

Here is a table of exercise precautions for individuals with specific health problems. If necessary, check with your doctor before you begin an exercise program.

Condition	Exercise Precautions
Arthritis	To reduce the stress on joints: 1. Begin all activity with an extensive warm-up to improve joint motion. Begin gently and progress gradually until you have increased the range of motion of your joints. 2. Select aerobic activities that minimize excessive stress on the afflicted joints. 3. Do not use hand or leg weights during aerobic activity. 4. Stop any exercise that causes significant pain.
Asthma	1. Begin with a gradual warm-up to reduce the risk of exercise-induced asthma (EIA). 2. If you use bronchodilator medications have them readily available in case EIA symptoms appear.

Condition	Exercise Precautions
Diabetes	1. Have digestible carbohydrates such as candy or fruit juice readily available in case you experience hypoglycemia. 2. Do not inject insulin into a muscle about to be used in exercise.
Coronary Heart Disease and Strokes	1. Maintain low to moderate intensities during aerobic exercise. 2. Check with your doctor to see whether your medication affects normal heart-rate response to exercise—if it does, you will have to use another method of monitoring exercise intensity besides taking your pulse.
Hypertension (high blood pressure)	1. Maintain low to moderate intensities during aerobic exercise. 2. Check with your doctor to see whether your medication affects normal heart-rate response to exercise—if it does, you will have to use another method of monitoring exercise intensity besides taking your pulse. 3. Avoid static strengthening exercise (isometrics). Isometric exercise involves forceful muscle activity against immovable objects, which results in elevated blood pressure. 4. Avoid exercising with your arms above your head for extended periods of time. 5. Avoid lifting excessively heavy weights. 6. When doing strength exercises, exhale on exertion (that is, during the time that the muscle is vigorously contracting).

Condition	Exercise Precautions
Joint Injury (such as runner's knee, tennis elbow)	1. Avoid exercises and activities that place undue stress on the affected joint.
Low Back Pain	1. Avoid use of hand or leg weights during aerobic activity. 2. Avoid movements such as high knee lifts, twisting the upper body, standing and bending forward in an unsupported position. 3. Stop any activity that causes back pain.
Pregnancy	1. Do not begin a vigorous exercise program at this time if you have not exercised regularly before becoming pregnant. 2. Avoid excessive pounding on your feet, because your joints are more lax during pregnancy. 3. After the fourth month, avoid exercising while lying on your back, to ensure that the weight of the baby will not obstruct the flow of blood back to your heart and head. 4. Maintain moderate intensities during aerobic activity. 5. Avoid stretching too far, because your joints are more lax during pregnancy.

If you smoke, you will probably find vigorous exercise more difficult than someone who does not. For your health's sake, why not expand your general goals to include quitting? Many people have found that the feeling of well-being that comes from a good exercise program helps them take control of other aspects of their lives. The new healthy you deserves only the best!

If you are significantly overweight, it is important that you avoid extremely stressful exercise and lose weight at a sensible rate. You should begin with a pre-aerobic program and gradually progress to a more vigorous program as you lose those unwanted pounds. In this way you can avoid injuries that can be caused by the extra weight that your bones and joints must support.

Postural Analysis

How many times did your parents or grandparents tell you to "stand up tall" or "sit up straight" when you were a child? You probably had no idea just how important this advice was at the time. Your posture affects the quality of your daily life. Many minor aches and pains can be attributed to poor posture, and so can the excruciating agony of severe low back pain. Many folks who seem to be injured more frequently than the average person have poor posture.

Unfortunately, as an adult, correcting posture is no longer as simple as following the good advice you were given as a child. Over the years you may have developed many unconscious and deeply ingrained habits that are reinforced by stiff joints and weak muscles. Whenever we lecture on this subject, we usually notice that many people in our audiences will immediately sit up straight as they become conscious about their lazy posture. But as soon as they become more relaxed, they inevitably begin to resume their habitual slump.

Poor posture can place an excessive burden on bones, joints, muscles, tendons, and ligaments. Even if you were never particularly uncomfortable before you began a vigorous exercise program, the abnormal stresses caused by faulty posture can result in injuries when you expose your body to the extra demands of a training program. Therefore, it is important to identify any significant postural imperfections that might predispose you to injuries, and it is also wise to avoid any demanding activities that are particularly threatening to people who have your deficiency.

A careful examination usually shows that one imperfection in posture is tied to a series of other postural abnormalities, because a change in body alignment in one part of the body requires that you compensate for the change in other areas to help maintain your balance. Improvements in posture can involve several different parts of the body, and no amount of effort at correcting only a single obvious misalignment will be successful. For example, someone who has round shoulders may be forced to arch the neck and stretch the chin forward in order to keep the head in an upright position. Effective treatment must include a series of complementary exercises for all affected parts of the body.

Here are some guidelines for taking the postural screening test:

- Wear a minimum of clothing, such as a bathing suit.
- Use a full-length mirror.
- Have someone help you with the side and rear views of your posture (ideally this should be someone who will also take part in the self-testing program). Alternatively, place two large mirrors at right angles to each other so you can see yourself in profile, or have someone take photographs or a video of you in profile and from the rear.
- Be sure to relax and assume your normal posture throughout the tests. It is tempting to stand the way we would like to be seen by others, rather than the way we stand when we are alone and fatigued.
- Use the checklist on the following pages. The table will tell you if your alignment is desirable or if you have postural imperfections. For each postural problem, a specific remedy will be suggested.

Body Part	Desirable	Imperfections
HEAD		Chin Forward

Remedy: This head position generally occurs as a compensation for round shoulders. Correcting round shoulders may help to properly realign the head.

Body Part	Desirable	Imperfections
UPPER BACK		Round Shoulders

Remedy: Stretch chest muscles (page 64) and strengthen muscles of the upper back (page 88).

Body Part	Desirable	Imperfections	
LOWER BACK		Arched Back	Flat Back

29

Remedy: For an arched back, stretch muscles of the hips (page 66), low back (page 65), and back of the thighs (page 68); strengthen the abdominals (page 89). For a flat back, seek medical attention.

Body Part	Desirable	Imperfections
ABDOMEN		Protruding Abdomen

Remedy: Stretch muscles of the low back (page 65); strengthen the abdominals (page 89).

Body Part	Desirable	Imperfections
KNEES		Hyperextended Knees

Remedy: Stretch the muscles on the front of the thighs (page 67); if the problem is severe hyperextension, seek medical advice before you take part in activities like running and aerobics.

Body Part	Desirable	Imperfections
FEET		High Arch

Remedy: Seek medical advice if you intend to take part in very vigorous activities where the feet strike the ground.

Body Part	Desirable	Imperfections
FEET		Morton's Foot

Remedy: The big toe is longer than the second toe in the normal foot. Morton's Foot is a fairly common inherited condition in which the second toe extends beyond the big toe. This tends to shift excessive weight on to the inner border of the foot. Over a period of time, especially in the physically active person, this will tend to flatten the arch of the foot. A qualified professional can provide arch supports that will help shift the weight away from the inner border of the foot.

31

Body Part	Desirable	Imperfections
SHOULDERS		Uneven Shoulders

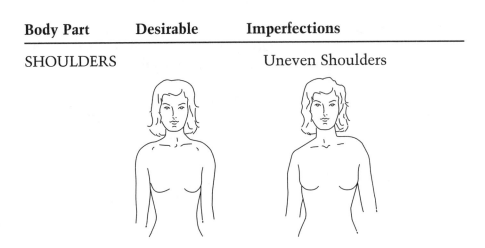

Remedy: This can be caused by carrying a heavy backpack or purse on one shoulder. Place your backpack across both shoulders or alternate your purse from side to side. If your hips and knees are also uneven, you should be evaluated by a medical expert.

Body Part	Desirable	Imperfections
HIPS		Uneven Hips

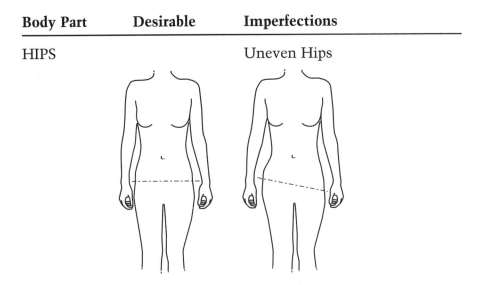

Remedy: If your shoulders and knees are also uneven, you should be evaluated by a medical expert.

Body Part	Desirable	Imperfections	
LEGS		Bowlegged	Knock-kneed

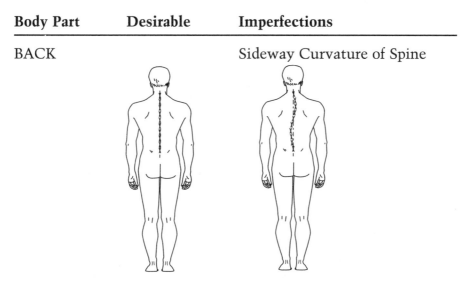

Remedy: Seek medical advice if you intend to participate in very vigorous activities where the feet strike the ground.

Body Part	Desirable	Imperfections
BACK		Sideway Curvature of Spine

Remedy: You have a condition known as scoliosis. An extremely mild sideways curvature of the spine may not create a problem during exercise, but an obvious sideways curvature should be evaluated by a medical expert.

Body Part	Desirable	Imperfections
FEET		Overpronation

Remedy: People who suffer from excessive pronation often have a flat-footed appearance. If in doubt, you should seek the advice of a specialist. Many people who have been fitted with custom-made corrective devices worn inside their shoes have been able to take part in frequent and vigorous exercise with no apparent problems. You will find it helpful to strengthen the intrinsic muscles of the feet (page 92).

Re-evaluate your posture every couple of months and remember that the muscles that maintain posture are used for many hours each day. If you're continually aware of your posture, you'll be able to make conscious adjustments that can eventually become habit.

Muscle Tightness Tests

Your lifestyle can create tightness in a number of your muscles. Some occupations involve continuous sitting or standing. Many factory assembly workers, cab drivers, bank tellers, and computer operators know all too well the aggravation that comes from nagging neck and low back pain. Continuous standing or sitting makes us tight in the muscles of the chest, the low back, the hips, and the calves. These conditions affect the natural alignment of the body. Poor body alignment places excessive stress on parts of the body that weren't designed for high levels of stress. The stress becomes even greater when a person decides to take up more vigorous physical activity. Therefore, it is important to test the tightness of your muscles and to engage in a regular stretching program to prevent muscles from becoming tight.

For purposes of good health, everyone should stretch regularly. But if the following tests indicate that you are overtight in some particular muscles, you should pay special attention to the exercises that will remedy your shortcoming. Appropriate corrective exercises should be selected from Chapter 5.

Here are instructions for taking the tests of muscle tightness:

- Dress lightly and comfortably.

- If it's convenient, find someone else who wishes to take the tests and assist each other. If you wish to do the tests by yourself, you will need to use a mirror to help you to examine a side view of your body positions.

- Put yourself into the body position required.

- Try to relax the rest of your body so that you consciously isolate the muscle being tested.

- Stretch the muscle as far as you can until you feel mild discomfort, not pain.

- Do not bounce or try to force yourself into the positions shown in the photographs.

- In each case, check to see whether you've achieved the "passing" criteria.

Test	Directions	Your Goal	Exercises (Chapter 5)
Shoulders	Reach backward and down to opposite shoulder blade	To touch top of shoulder blade	Elbow press Overarm shoulder press

35

Test	Directions	Your Goal	**Exercises** (Chapter 5)
Shoulders	Reach backward and up to opposite shoulder blade	To touch bottomof shoulder blade	Underarm shoulder press
Lower Back	Lying on your back, pull both knees toward chest	Knees should touch chest	Knees to chest
Front of Hips	Lying on your back, pull one knee to chest, other leg fully extended on floor	Calf of extended leg must remain on floor; knee must not bend	Hip stretches

36

Test	Directions	Your Goal	**Exercises** (Chapter 5)
Back of thighs	Lying on your back, lift one leg, keeping other leg flat on the floor, without bending either knee	Raised leg must must reach a vertical position	Hamstring stretches
Front of thighs	Lying on your stomach with the knees together, gently pull heel toward buttocks	Heel should comfortably touch buttocks	Quadriceps stretch
Calves	Standing with your back, buttocks, and heels against a wall, raise one forefoot up off the floor, keeping both knees straight but relaxed and heels down	Ball of foot should clear floor by at least the width of two fingers	Wall press Hurdle stretch

Repeat these tests every month to monitor your progress. Once you can pass the tests, continue to do the stretches regularly to prevent muscle tightness from reoccuring.

Muscle Strength Tests

Even though you may lead a busy and physically active life, some of your muscles are probably not being used as much as is desirable for good health and fitness. While your lower back muscles may tend to be strong—as a result of the constant need to counteract the downward pull of gravity—the opposing muscles in your abdomen become weak from disuse. That's why almost everyone should do regular strengthening exercises for the abdominals. The millions of Americans who have protruding abdomens are walking (or usually sitting) examples of the results of this imbalance. You can utilize many of your neglected muscles during daily activities by conditioning yourself to deliberately use them until it becomes second nature. Round shoulders can be avoided, for example, if you first stretch the tight muscles of the chest and then consciously pull the shoulders back.

Measuring muscle strength as it relates to health is very difficult without elaborate equipment. Although there are many strength tests such as those that measure how many sit-ups and push-ups you can perform in a specific amount of time, these tests tend to evaluate not one but several factors combined: the endurance of your muscles (the ability of the muscle to do many repetitions); your strength; the skill required to perform the task. These tests measure your performance as it compares to "norms." That is, your score is compared with the scores of large numbers of people who have taken the same test in the past. What these tests don't tell you is how many repetitions or how much strength you need to avoid problems that contribute to injury and discomfort.

Much more important in reducing the risk of pain and injury is the relative strength of your muscles. For example, if your low back muscles are stronger than the abdominals or if your calf muscles are stronger than the muscles on the front of the shin, then you have a muscle imbalance. No matter how weak or strong you are, you may have a muscle imbalance if the muscles on one side of the joint are stronger than the muscles on the other side of the joint. Only sophisticated clinical or research equipment can accurately estimate the relative strength of opposing muscle groups.

However, there is an excellent test that you can use to test the relative strength of two of the most important groups of muscles in your body. These muscles are your abdominals and also a pair of powerful groin muscles that pull your thighs towards your chest. These latter muscles are called the iliacus and psoas. The relative strength of these two muscle groups is a good indicator of your likelihood of suffering from low back pain. When you are standing, your abdominals tend to flatten your lower back, but your left and right psoas muscles will tend to arch your lower back. If your psoas muscles are much tighter and stronger than your abdominals your back will tend to be excessively arched. This puts uneven compression on the spine and often leads to nagging back ache. If you have a history of back pain, this test is unnecessary, and you may find it painful, so you should not try it without medical approval. If you do not suffer from low back pain, this test is a safe and effective way to assess the relative strength of two important groups of muscles.

Lie on your back and stretch your legs to a vertical position, as shown in Figure 3-1. Flatten your lower back firmly against the floor. Very slowly, lower your legs as shown, and try to keep your lower back flattened against the floor surface for as long as you possibly can. When your back arches off the floor, as shown in Figure 3-2, the test is complete. For safety's sake, bend your knees and lower your feet to the floor. We recommend that you perform the test with a partner and have him or her ready to support the weight of your legs when your low back begins to arch off the floor. Your partner can also check how far you can lower your legs before your back arches, or alternatively, lay parallel with a full length mirror and look at your own reflection. Compare your results with this scale.

Less than 30 degrees from the vertical	= Poor
30 degrees from the vertical (Figure 3-3)	= Fair
60 degrees from the vertical (Figure 3-4)	= Good
Within 15 degrees of horizontal (Figure 3-5)	= Excellent
All the way to the floor	= Superb

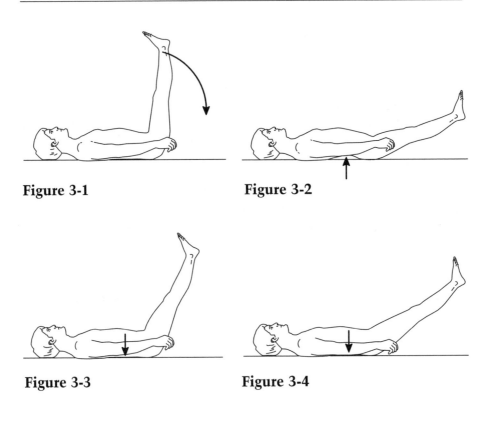

Figure 3-1   **Figure 3-2**

Figure 3-3   **Figure 3-4**

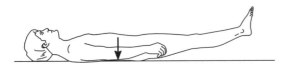

Figure 3-5

Most people do not do well on this test, and so almost everyone can benefit from the abdominal strengthening exercises described in Chapter 6.

As it is unlikely that you'll have the opportunity to test your strength with elaborate equipment, we offer you general guidelines to help you deal with potential muscle weaknesses. Since the abdominal and shin muscles are rarely used in the course of a normal day, they tend to be weaker than their opposing muscle groups. This may not create a problem for most inactive individuals, because the body is not being excessively stressed. Once you decide to become more active, however, these forms of muscle imbalance can result in excessive stress being placed on the body, which can in turn result in pain or injury. We therefore recommend that inactive individuals perform abdominal and shin strength exercises (page 89 and 91). If you detect that you are round-shouldered, we also recommend that you do upper back strength exercises (page 88).

You should also be concerned about the absolute strength of your muscles. A minimum level of strength is necessary to ensure that you can meet the demand of everyday living. You should seek expert advice if you realize that you are particularly weak in important muscle groups. As a general guide, if you are unable to maintain good postural alignment of your abdominal and low back region without a conscious effort and you suffer from more than occasional low back pain, your abdominals need special attention. If you find that 10 to 15 toe taps (page 91) create significant discomfort in the muscle on the front of your shins, then these muscles need to be strengthened. Finally, remember that traditional calisthenics such as push-ups and chins are not appropriate for everyone. Learn to be a discriminating exerciser. Every strengthening exercise that you do should be done for some intelligent purpose.

Aerobic Fitness Test

The most effective way of testing your aerobic fitness requires elaborate equipment and trained professionals to administer an appropriate testing procedure. Accurate testing of this kind may be unnecessary and perhaps too costly for many people. However, as your fitness is determined by the amount of vigorous activity you do, it is possible for you to obtain an estimate of your present aerobic fitness from nothing more than your answers to three simple questions: In a typical week, how hard do you exercise? How long do you exercise? How often do you exercise? The simple test that follows has been developed from previous tests as a result of recent research that has established how much aerobic exercise a person needs to do to be considered healthy.

The purpose of this test is to help you determine the best level for you to begin or continue a program of aerobic exercise. This is particularly important for two reasons. First, you obviously want to do enough exercise to get some health benefits. On the other hand, you want to avoid pain and injuries. Many injuries seem to occur when people try to do too much too soon.

Directions: Locate the phrase that best describes the intensity of your normal weekly physical activity and circle the number that corresponds to that category. Similarly, circle the numbers that correspond to the duration and frequency of your normal weekly physical activity. Multiply the three circled numbers together (intensity times duration times frequency). Locate your score on the table, which will indicate your approximate aerobic fitness level and tell you the point at which you should begin your exercise program. Here is an example. Suppose you exercise four days per week for 20 minutes each session at a moderate pace. You would score 3 points for frequency, 3 points for duration, and 4 points for intensity for a total score of $3 \times 3 \times 4 = 36$. According to the chart that follows, a score of 36 represents a fitness level that is "good" and you can begin aerobic exercise program at an "intermediate level."

Frequency	Score
Daily	5
5 to 6 times a week	4
3 to 4 times a week	3
1 to 2 times a week	2
Less than once a week	1

Duration of Continuous Activity	Score
Over 30 minutes (continuous activity)	5
21 to 30 minutes	4
11 to 20 minutes	3
6 to 10 minutes	2
under 5 minutes	1

Intensity	Score
Sustained heavy breathing (examples: highly skilled runner, bicyclist, swimmer, dancer, or power walker)	5
Sustained moderate breathing (examples: skilled runner, bicyclist, swimmer, dancer, power walker)	4
or	
Intermittent heavy breathing (examples: highly skilled player of raquetball, tennis, or basketball}	
Intermittent moderate breathing (examples: less skilled player of racquetball, tennis, or basketball)	3
Light breathing (examples: leisurely walking, cycling, swimming, or dancing)	2
Normal breathing (examples: resting state while sitting or standing)	1

Score	Fitness Level	Starting Point
64 and above	High—very active	Advanced
36 to 63	Good—active	Intermediate
18 to 35	Fair—mildly active	Beginner
9 to 17	Poor—barely active	Maintenance pre-aerobic
8 and under	Very poor—not active	Pre-aerobic program

Retest your aerobic fitness level every few months.

We cannot overemphasize the fact that you can avoid pain and injuries by starting an aerobic fitness program at a level that your body can handle and by avoiding sudden increases in the amount of aerobic activity you do.

Most aerobic exercise-related injuries result from impatience, unrestrained optimism, or a lack of understanding about the way the body adapts to sudden increases in exercise. This applies not only to beginners but to people who have been performing an activity at one level for some time and then suddenly decide to exercise more vigorously for longer periods of time. Some years back when we were both less well-informed, we made the mistake of increasing our exercise regimens too drastically. For a long time Lorna would run 2 to 3 miles every other day. Then one summer she was bitten by the running bug. Within two weeks she increased her mileage so that she was doing as much as 35 to 40 miles a week. After moving from the flatlands of Ames, Iowa, to the challenging hills of Eugene, Oregon, Peter made the mistake of attempting to maintain the same weekly cycling mileage on a much more challenging course. As a result of trying to do too much too soon, Lorna suffered from hip pain for some time and Peter had to stop cycling for several weeks until his Achilles tendinitis cleared up. Both of us made the mistake of greatly increasing the amount of exercise that we were doing without allowing our musculoskeletal systems time to adapt to the added stress on our bodies.

Research has shown that exercise can increase the resilience of all of the components of the musculoskeletal system. These structures are the muscles, bones, joints, tendons, and ligaments. Improvements in the resilience of these components will in turn reduce the chance of injury. Improvements do not occur immediately, however, and the rate of change varies from one component to the next. If you are patient and do not increase the amount of exercise faster than the rate at which these important anatomical structures can become more resilient, you will reduce your chances of becoming hurt.

In many instances people don't know how much activity they should start with. Generally, the better your aerobic fitness level within an activity, the more activity you can do. Notice we said "within an activity." You may be a very fit runner but an unfit cyclist. Do not assume that your fitness level encompasses every activity.

Now that you have completed the self-tests, you have learned enough about your unique body to be able to begin to design a personalized program that is exactly right for you. The next step is to make certain that the activities and exercises you will choose to help you meet your exercise goals are the right ones.

If the results of our tests appear to indicate that you're likely to have a problem, the following options are available to you:

1. In many cases you can begin a specific program of stretching and strengthening exercises to improve certain deficiencies. If you are round-shouldered, for example, we recommend that you do exercises that stretch your chest muscles and other exercises that strengthen the muscles of your upper back. Specific exercises are discussed in Chapters 5 and 6.

2. We recommend that you seek medical attention for obvious deficiencies that can't be readily corrected with stretching and strengthening exercises. We come back to the example of Jeff, the flat-footed cyclist. With the aid of a relatively inexpensive, nonsurgical treatment, the medical specialist was able to help Jeff overcome a problem that had caused him a great deal of pain. In other instances an expert can reassure you that an apparent problem indicated by the simple tests is no cause for concern. In the latter case the old adage "Better safe than sorry" would seem to be a wise one.

3. If you have an obvious deficiency but choose not to seek medical advice, you should attempt to avoid forms of exercise that are known to be especially stressful to someone with your deficiency. For example, people who have a marked curvature of the lower back (lumbar lordosis) may be susceptible to pain and injuries if they run long distances, whereas the same people are usually pain and injury-free if they swim instead.

FIT TIPS

1. You can reduce your risk of becoming injured by correcting any structural problems you might have and by avoiding sudden increases in the amount of exercise you do.

2. Use the self-tests to record your health history and to evaluate your posture, flexibility, and strength.

3. Take the Aerobic Fitness Test to find your present aerobic fitness level.

4. Use the results of the tests to help you select exercises for your own personalized exercise program.

Chapter 4

CHOOSING DISCRIMINATE EXERCISES AND ACTIVITIES

A common misconception surrounding exercise is that *any* form of exercise is good for you. Put another way, most people seem to believe that if you take part in *any* fitness activity or perform *any* type of calisthenic exercise, you will automatically improve your health and well-being. Not so. In order to be safe and effective, each and every activity or exercise that you include in an exercise program should be done for a specific reason.

Look around whenever you are among a group of people taking part in informal exercise. Watch people on the beach or at the park. Typically, you will see a few assorted stretches, including toe touching, side bends, and arm circling, as well as a random selection of popular strengthening exercises, including push-ups and sit-ups. Few people can give specific reasons for doing any of the calisthenic rituals they perform, but they will usually tell you they have done these things ever since they were in school. One of the most common reasons people give for taking part in popular

47

exercise activities such as running, aerobic dance, swimming, cycling, and weight training is that "everyone seems to be doing it." We refer to this kind of haphazard and arbitrary exercise behavior as *indiscriminate* participation. Indiscriminate participation takes two forms. Many people are indiscriminate about the physical activities they choose, and those same people are often indiscriminate about the exercises they perform before, during, and after their chosen exercise activities.

Indiscriminate activities are often performed when an individual randomly chooses a form of exercise in the hope that it might do some good. Greg, for example, had just passed his 40th birthday and was a little sensitive to his wife's humorous comments about his expanding paunch, so he decided to start a fitness program. He headed to a nearby health club and began regular sessions in the weight training room. After three months, Greg complained to us that his body was just the same as when he had started and he was suffering from frequent bouts of low back pain. We first asked him what his exercise goals were. He said that he wanted to "lose some weight, firm up my muscles, and become a bit more limber." He also mentioned that his father had suffered a heart attack at a relatively early age and he wanted to improve his own cardiovascular condition.

Greg seemed stunned when we told him that weight training was not the best way to achieve all of his goals. Although systematic weight training can increase your metabolism (which in turn can lead to improved body composition), conventional weight training has little or no effect on the heart and lungs, and so it is not an effective way to reduce the risk of heart disease. Even worse, incorrectly executed weight training exercises can damage the musculoskeletal system. Greg obviously made an indiscriminate choice when he decided to work with weights as a way of attaining his exercise goals.

There are probably millions of Americans who have exercise goals similar to Greg's. Perhaps he reminds you of someone you know. When you've finished this book, you'll be able to help that person design a personalized exercise program to reach his or her own special exercise goals. Especially if that person is you.

Indiscriminate exercises are used by people who perform stretching and strengthening calisthenics at random as part of a training program. Ever since people became aware that exercise could affect their ability to perform strenuous tasks, they have devised stretching and strengthening exercises to prepare them for various forms of combat and athletic competition. At some time in the distant past, various exercises such as push-ups, sit-ups, chinning, knee bends, and toe touching became commonly used. In recent years, a scientific procedure known as electromyography has allowed us to examine these exercises in detail and to understand their actual effects on the muscles. Unfortunately, the vast majority of people who routinely perform these traditional exercises have superficial, and frequently erroneous, ideas about their effects. In the folklore of fitness, these kinds of calisthenics are deemed essential for *all* exercise programs. This indiscriminate approach to exercise is based on the assumption that traditional exercises are the cure for just about any fitness problem the body might have.

But let's get back to Greg. We asked him why he routinely did an exercise known as a bench press, which involves pushing a weight up toward the ceiling and lowering it back toward the chest while you lie on your back. Greg said it was "for my pecs (chest muscles) and triceps." When we asked him why these muscles needed to be strengthened, he seemed at a loss. Likewise, he seemed to believe that an exercise which involved lifting his feet from the floor while he was lying flat on his back with his legs straight (leg lifts, page 95) was good for his stomach muscles, and that this in turn would "get rid of the fat around my midriff." But this exercise does not effectively strengthen the abdominal nor does it selectively remove fat from the belly. In fact, this exercise is exceptionally stressful to the low back and can cause discomfort and injury to this vulnerable region.

In his other endeavors Greg is an obviously intelligent person. His professional life as a lawyer revolves around searching for verifiable facts. Yet he told us that his information about weight training came from "the guys around the gym." Unfortunately, experience has shown that Greg's approach to exercise is the rule, not the exception.

Many people who work out informally at home also use indiscriminate exercises. Carl proudly told one of his professors, "I am a real exercise nut. Every single morning I roll out of bed and do 75 push-ups." Carl, who has very poor posture, was obviously unaware that frequent push-ups can actually contribute to a round-shouldered appearance. Indiscriminate stretching exercises can also be counterproductive. Many gymnasts and dancers try to maintain flexibility by regularly touching their toes without bending at the knees. Unfortunately, this exercise can actually produce a permanent hyperextension of the knees (knees pushed backwards), making the knee joints more vulnerable to injuries.

These examples point to the importance of doing every exercise for a specific reason. We call this *discriminate exercise.* You should also select activities that will accomplish precisely what you want to achieve in your exercise program. We call these *discriminate activities.* If you don't know precisely what any particular exercise is doing for you, stop doing it until you find out. Indiscriminate exercise may be potentially harmful, and indiscriminate activities may not allow you to achieve what you want to from your exercise program.

Here's an example of a discriminate activity used to meet a SMART goal. (Remember: SMART is an acronym for Specific, Measurable, Action-oriented, Realistic, and Timed.) This example also illustrates how discriminate exercises are an essential part of any discriminate activity. Members of many of the teams that will represent the United States in the 1996 Summer Olympic Games in Atlanta have been in continuous training since 1992. Each team member has had one or more specific goals that he or she is striving to achieve. Examples of these goals include throwing farther, jumping higher, or running faster. With the assistance of coaches and trainers, progress has been measured at regular intervals. Therefore, each goal was action-oriented because the individual athlete had a carefully devised plan to improve performance. Each goal was also discriminate because the athletes have used scientifically-proven techniques to help them to improve performance.

For a number of years, Peter has worked with Olympic volleyball, cycling, and synchronized swimming teams, and with many of the world's best water-skiers. In each case, he carried out a personalized fitness assessment using similar tests to those described in Chapter 3. Surprisingly, the results of the tests showed that some very successful athletes were actually inflexible in specific joints, and relatively weak in one or more of the muscles groups that are important for the performance of the athlete's specific sport.

For example, it was readily apparent that the jumping performance of a number of world-class volleyball players and water-ski jumpers was restricted by a combination of a lack of strength and inflexibility in the low back and legs. Also, the specific muscles and joints involved varied from athlete to athlete. On the basis of the results of the fitness assessment tests and other available data, individualized sets of specific strength training and complementary stretching exercises were given to each athlete.

Research has shown that specific kinds of weight training and an advanced training technique known as "Plyometrics" are extremely effective ways to strengthen the muscles used in jumping. Weight training and plyometrics were, therefore, discriminate choices of activities. A variety of machines and free weights were used to ensure that each exercise strengthened the specific muscles involved in jumping, with special emphasis being given to the individual athlete's weakest muscles. Plyometric training which involves "rebounding" or forceful stretching of the muscles immediately before jumping is mechanically stressful on the body, so it was not used until it became apparent that the individual had sufficient strength to withstand the rigors of this advanced technique.

To ensure that all exercises were done correctly, experienced trainers carefully monitored each athlete's training program. The results confirmed that the goal of improving jumping ability with specific weight training exercises was realistic. Finally, the goal of each athlete was timed. Every member of the two teams had a burning desire to be at the peak of his or her jumping ability at precisely the right time—the start of the competition in the Olympic games for the volleyball players, and the world championships for the water-ski jumpers.

Choosing the Right Clothing and Equipment

Exercise often involves the use of equipment, and this is another area where you should make discriminate choices. Basically, exercise equipment falls into three categories: clothing, footwear, and hardware. As a general rule it is wise to seek the advice of experts in each area before you make selections, but here are a few simple considerations that can help you to make discriminate choices.

Clothing

Exercise and sports clothing is a major segment of the fashion market, so most people can find clothing to suit their budget and their tastes. Clothing has two important roles to play in your exercise program: optimizing body temperature during exercise and protecting the body from injury.

Clothing can prevent heat loss in cold weather. In severe winter conditions some joggers, walkers, cyclists, and cross-country skiers wear thermal underwear, insulated outerwear, and gloves. Swimmers can prolong their swimming program during colder months by wearing a snug-fitting neoprene wet suit. But because strenuous exercise a will markedly raise your body temperature, there are many occasions a when you will want to lose heat rather than retain it. Loose-fitting clothes made from fabrics that allow water vapor to pass freely are ideally suited to this purpose. For some time the trend has been away from synthetics like nylon that form an insulated barrier which retards heat loss. Instead, many experienced exercise enthusiasts have turned to natural, breathable fabrics like cotton. Textile technology has recently produced synthetic products that have the durability of nylon and the permeability of cotton. The simple rule for losing heat, however, is to wear as little as possible so that perspiration on the skin is exposed to the movement of the surrounding air.

In activities requiring the full range of motion of the joints, particularly stretching and strengthening exercises, it is important that clothing not restrict free movement. On the other hand, you should be aware that baggy garments could become entangled in moving parts of machines such as those used for weight training and cycling.

The protective role of clothing is an important consideration for activities that pose a risk of tripping and falling. Cycling or in-line skating in your swimsuit may be "cool" in more ways than one, but uncovered elbows and knees are particularly vulnerable in a fall. And remember that your head is the only one you will ever have, so wear a protective helmet at all times. Clothing also provides effective protection against excessive exposure to the sun. Sunburn can be painful, and dermatologists have warned that people who undergo repeated and prolonged exposure to the sun greatly increase their chances of getting skin cancer.

Footwear

One of the most common questions we are asked when we lecture about any particular exercise activity is "What is the best shoe for this activity?" Experience has shown us that many people want us to say that "Model X" is *the* best shoe for *everyone!* Unfortunately, our advice is not so simple. The most logical way to make a discriminate choice of exercise footwear is to ask yourself two simple questions: "What am I going to use them for?" and "What kind of shoes do my feet need?"

Many shoes are designed to improve your athletic performance, but the primary purpose of shoes is to protect you from injury. Activities involving repeated pounding of your feet against a firm surface can subject your body to stresses that may cause a variety of injuries. Shoes designed for walking, running, aerobics, and various court sports have a substantial layer of shock-absorbing material sandwiched between your foot and the outer sole of the shoe to cushion these impacts.

Runners and walkers usually strike the ground with the heel first, so running and walking shoes must have adequate cushioning under the heel. For aerobics and court sports, adequate cushioning under the ball of the foot is important. Cyclists are not subjected to repeated impacts, so their shoes don't require cushioning. Bicycle touring can involve both cycling and walking, so you should look for a shoe that will provide fairly good rigidity and some cushioning.

A shoe must also provide the correct amount of traction on the surface it will be used on. Runners and walkers move almost exclusively in a forward direction, and it is important for them to avoid slipping and sliding. Consequently, running and walking shoes must have a roughened outsole that will grip the surface of the ground. Many different outsole designs will effectively provide a high level of traction on concrete and asphalt. If you exercise on other surfaces, however, such as wet grass or sand, you may find that some outsoles are more effective than others. Quite simply, you should run or walk cautiously the first time you wear a new type of shoe or try a track or trail for the first time. The salespeople who work in stores that specialize in exercise and sports footwear are usually familiar with local jogging and walking trails and they will probably be pleased to offer you some advice. Don't be afraid to take back any shoes that do not live up to the promises made by the salesperson, however.

Activities like aerobics and court sports require a moderately high level of traction, because they involve continual changes in direction, back and forth and side to side. To avoid abrupt, stressful impacts when you make these directional changes, your feet must be able to slide for a short distance just after each foot strikes the ground. Human beings do this best when they land on the ball of the foot, so the tread pattern on this area of the outsole is an important design feature.

Finally, footwear can play another important role in making exercise as safe as possible. Clinical examinations have shown that a relatively large proportion of the population have imperfect feet. In particular, many people suffer from a condition that runners call *overpronation*, shown on page 34. This condition results from a variety of factors, including a lack of muscle tone, stretched ligaments, misshapen bones in the feet, and above all, genetic factors. People who overpronate tend to support their weight on the inner side of the feet, especially when they perform vigorous activities like running and jumping. Overpronation tends to put additional stress on the knee joints and shins, which can eventually lead to pain and injuries. It can often be corrected with custom-made orthotic that fits unobtrusively inside each shoe.

Overpronators usually have a flat-footed appearance, but it generally takes a trained expert to actually diagnose the severity of this condition. Anyone who appears to overpronate is advised to see a sports-medicine specialist. Fortunately, people who tend to overpronate can also get some help from well-designed shoes.

The ability of a shoe to restrict the amount of pronation is sometimes called "motion control." A lightweight shoe made from flimsy materials, such as a ballet slipper, will simply change its shape with the movements of the foot. But shoe technologists have been able to modify different parts of a shoe so that it can effectively act as a splint whenever your foot tends to roll excessively inward or outward. For running, walking, aerobics, cross-country skiing, and court sports, the sole of the shoe must remain flexible round the ball of the foot so that you will not be restricted when you lift your heels up from the ground. When you cycle, the shape of your foot does not change appreciably, so cycling shoes are deliberately inflexible. Weight training can expose your feet to extremely high forces, so suitable footwear should provide good motion control.

Some people actually pronate less than normal (sometimes called "underpronation") because they tend to have fairly rigid and in many cases high-arched feet. Motion control isn't a concern for these individuals, but the rigidity of their feet makes them especially susceptible to injury from impact shock, so they should be especially careful to choose shoes that provide good cushioning.

Quite clearly, each exercise activity has unique footwear requirements and, as a result of technological advances, manufacturers can now provide shoes for the activity of your choice. For very dissimilar activities the best protection will be provided by different types of shoes. It is unlikely that you would be tempted to use stiff cycling shoes for a jogging program. On the other hand, a number of fitness enthusiasts who do not specialize exclusively in any one activity find that a well-designed shoe that has good overall cushioning and good motion control can be used for a number of purposes. Because this kind of shoe has to serve different functions, it is referred to as a cross-training shoe, and is usually a little more robust than some of the lighter single-activity shoes.

The first factor you should consider in choosing footwear for exercise will be the activity or activities you intend to perform in your exercise program. The next consideration is your own unique feet. Without a doubt, the most crucial aspect of a shoe is fit. The best designed shoe in the world cannot provide you with the cushioning, traction, and motion control that you need if it doesn't fit!

Different shoes are constructed around different *lasts,* which are rigid devices that are shaped like a human foot. The shoe you need is the shoe that was built on a last that looks just like your foot. Your foot should fit snugly in both the front and back of the shoe, but podiatrists recommend that you have about a half-inch of space between your big toe and the inside of the toe of the shoe. This prevents your toes from bumping against the end of the shoe when you make sudden stops.

Exercise Hardware

Most pieces of hardware can be classified as devices either to increase strength or to improve aerobic fitness. Strength training equipment will be discussed in Chapter 6 and aerobic training devices will be discussed in Chapter 8. The major considerations in making discriminate choices of hardware are first safety and then effectiveness.

Unfortunately, TV shopping channels feature new exercise machines every other week. Remember that few of these gadgets have ever been subjected to careful scientific evaluation, and the long-term effects of using them has not been determined. For safety's sake, you should be familiar with the *purpose* of any machine you use. You should also take the time to inspect it periodically, since any device that has moving parts is susceptible to breakage. Remember to adjust machines such as weight training devices that use springs, pulleys, and cams, as well as aerobic exercise machines like bicycles (including stationary bikes), rowing machines, and skiing simulators to your unique body dimensions. If you feel stress in parts of your body that should not be stressed by the device, seek expert advice. But remember that you are the best judge of your own comfort. Now that you have learned the value of discriminate exercises, choose only those fitness aids that are safe and appropriate for reaching your specific exercise objectives.

In summary, you are faced with a series of choices when you are formulating the action plan to meet your unique exercise goals. *Discriminate* activities and exercises will help you reach your goals and achieve specific changes in those components of fitness that you wish to change, while *discriminate* choices of clothes, footwear, and hardware will enhance the safety and effectiveness of your exercise program.

FIT TIPS

1. Be a "discriminating exerciser": Choose exercises and physical activities that are right for your body and meet your own unique exercise goals.

2. Know what you are doing, and why you are doing it! Stretch or strengthen for a purpose, and choose aerobic activities that are right for you.

3. Avoid unsafe exercise positions.

4. Make discriminate choices about the exercise clothes, shoes, and equipment you select.

5. Make sure your exercise clothing allows you freedom of movement and helps keep your body at the right temperature.

6. Choose comfortable shoes that meet the needs of your unique feet *and* the activity you will be performing. If you have flat feet, you will probably need a broader fitting shoe that will also control side-to-side movements of your feet. If you have high-arched feet, you will probably need a shoe that provides extra cushioning.

Chapter 5

HOW TO STRETCH YOUR MUSCLES

Many people overlook the importance of stretching or regard it as a waste of time. In fact, it is one of the most important forms of exercise you can do. Any muscle that is not stretched frequently, either by your ordinary daily activities or by specific stretching exercises, will become shorter and tighter. This is particularly true of those muscles whose *strength* is continually maintained by everyday activities. For example, the hamstring muscles on the back of the thighs are strengthened by normal walking, running, and stair climbing. However, while the hamstring muscles are strengthened through daily activity, few people do anything on a daily basis to stretch these tight muscles. As a result, the hamstrings are susceptible to injury in many unfit people. Any sudden stretch that tends to forcibly extend them beyond their shortened limits can produce a painful torn muscle. A good example is the beginner aerobic dancer, motivated by the exciting beat of the music, who vigorously kicks her leg above her waist and ends up with a painful tear in her hamstring muscle.

Stretching in general is important for several reasons:

1. *Stretching can maintain or improve your appearance by ensuring good posture.* People who sit for long periods of

time can develop a round-shouldered posture if their chest muscles are not stretched regularly. In the same way, stretching tight low back muscles can reduce the tendency to stand in a swayback posture with your abdomen protruding.

2. *Stretching can improve your efficiency in sports and daily activities.* A swimmer who has tight shoulder muscles will have trouble doing the front crawl effectively. Without good shoulder flexibility it is almost impossible to lift the hands and elbows out of the water at the end of each arm stroke. Dragging them forward through the water reduces swimming speed and causes early fatigue. Good flexibility offers everyday benefits as well. It can help you reach just a little farther and higher as you retrieve items from cupboards and shelves. A stretching program could also improve your ability to perform tasks in restricted spaces when you work on your car or in your workplace.

3. *Stretching can reduce the risk of exercise-related injury and pain.* Inflexible people often put excessive stresses on inappropriate parts of the body. A good example is the tennis player who cannot turn sideways to serve the ball because the shoulder muscles are too tight. This clumsy and inefficient action can put stress on the elbow and may be one of the causes of "tennis elbow." Have you ever seen people who walk with a spring in their step? You probably thought they were happy-go-lucky individuals bounding through life. Guess again! They probably have tight calf muscles and are unable to keep their heels down on the ground for as long as a flexible person can. This bouncy walking pattern can become a problem when these people take to jogging, because tight calf muscles can force them to land on the balls of their feet, rather than on their heels, which can adversely affect the body's natural shock-absorbing mechanism.

Muscles that are too tight can also put pressure on sensitive parts of the body, causing years of pain and suffering. For example, tight hip flexors (the muscles that pull the thigh toward the chest) and tight lower back muscles are probably the primary causes of low back pain.

These problems can be easily resolved by spending a few minutes every day stretching the appropriate muscles. The appealing aspect of stretching is that it requires no special equipment or setting.

Stretching Dos and Don'ts

1. DO wear clothing that is comfortable and nonbinding.

2. DO warm up carefully before stretching. Perform some gentle activity that uses many of the large muscles of the body, such as walking or easy jogging in place while gently swinging the arms. This raises the temperature of the muscles slightly and lubricates the joints, making stretching more comfortable and effective.

3. DO select a body position that is most comfortable for you. Because of our unique genetic makeup, some of us have joints that are inherently more or less flexible than others. You should select stretching exercises that your own individual body will allow you to perform comfortably. Whenever possible, we will provide you with alternative exercises that will accomplish the same goal. Choose the ones that are most practical for you.

4. DO stretch to the point where you feel *mild* tension in the muscle, and hold each stretch for 10 to 30 seconds.

5. DON'T stretch to the point of pain. Pain is the body's way of telling you something could be wrong. You are probably exceeding the limits of the muscle and may actually be doing damage. With practice, you will learn to listen to your body so that you can tell the difference between mild discomfort and pain.

6. DON'T bounce. When you bounce up and down or back and forth in an effort to stretch a muscle, a reflex mechanism will tighten the very muscle you are trying to

stretch. Healthy muscles try to protect themselves from damage by forcefully contracting when they are suddenly stretched. This can cause tiny tears inside the muscles and will result in greater muscle soreness the following day. If you like to exercise to music, select tunes that DON'T have a strong beat. This will help you avoid the temptation to bounce.

7. DO isolate and stretch one muscle group at a time. If you stretch more than one muscle group at the same time, you can't be sure which specific muscle is the tightest and needs the most work. You will not be able to monitor progress this way. General exercises such as toe touching tend to stretch so the low back, as well as the back of the thighs and sometimes the calves (depending on your body position). It would be more effective to stretch one of these muscle groups at a time, being sure that each muscle is able to stretch to a healthy length.

8. DON'T stretch in ways that will force the joints beyond their normal ranges of motion. Pressing a joint forcefully into a locked position stretches the protective ligaments and weakens the joint. Gymnastics, some yoga positions, and classical ballet require an abnormal range of motion of some joints. If you are involved in these activities, you should carefully consider the long-term effects of creating this condition, which is known as *hypermobility.* Seek the guidance of an expert whose interest is in your safety and long-term well-being.

9. DO stretch on as many days a week as you can, preferably every day. The more frequently you stretch, the more likely you are to avoid tight muscles.

10. DO be patient. It may have taken months or even years for some muscles to become as tight as they are, so it will take some time to gradually restore them to their normal lengths.

11. DON'T do any exercise if at any time you experience pain or severe discomfort. Not every exercise is right for

everyone. For example, the front of the thigh stretch (see photo on page 68) is not appropriate for the person who has had recent knee surgery. See a medical expert if you feel any unusual pain.

Stretching Exercises

It is possible to stretch each and every one of the major muscles of your body, but some muscles need more attention than others. It is especially important to stretch those muscles that are necessary to maintain general fitness and good posture, and we will remind you about those that are essential in preparing you for specific aerobic activities. The stretches that follow are designed to reduce the risk of injury and are suitable for almost everyone.

Remember that the main purpose of this book is to help you achieve a level of overall fitness that will prepare you to take part in vigorous activities of your choice. If you are interested in becoming highly proficient in an activity that requires exceptional flexibility, this book will help you build a foundation for your goals. These specialized activities require you to stretch beyond what is considered normal limits, however, and you should consult another book or expert in the specific area that interests you.

In the following section we'll identify the area of the body to be stretched, explain the importance for stretching the muscles involved, and finally offer you a series of alternative stretches. Whenever possible, we'll give you the choice of doing each stretching exercise in a standing, sitting, or lying position so you can select the position most comfortable for you or the one that suits your particular circumstance. If you are outside and about to run in your new workout clothes, for example, you may prefer to stretch standing up rather than lying down on the ground.

If at any time you experience severe pain or discomfort, stop doing the exercise. Many of these exercises are intended for both sides of the body, but for the sake of brevity we illustrate them only on the left or right side. When it is appropriate, you should repeat the stretch for both sides.

Shoulders

Purpose: To relieve tightness in the shoulders that results from lazy posture while performing daily activities such as sitting at a desk or the wheel of a car. Shoulder tightness is the reason many people find it difficult to effectively perform overarm movements in such activities as tennis, swimming, or throwing a ball.

Exercise: *Elbow press.* Stand with your feet shoulder-width apart, knees relaxed, chest up and shoulders back. Place your hand behind your head and reach for the opposite shoulder blade. Using your other hand, push gently down on the raised elbow until you feel mild tightness.

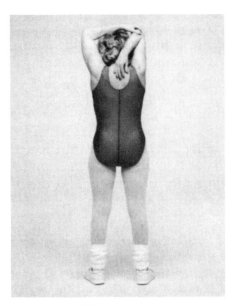

Elbow press.

Chest

Purpose: To correct the round shoulders people tend to develop through lazy posture while sitting and standing, which can adversely affect their mechanics when they exercise.

Exercises: *Overhead shoulder press.* Stand with your feet shoulder-width apart, knees relaxed, chest up and shoulders back. Grasp your hands above the head and bend the elbows. Gently push the arms backward. Do not arch the back. This exercise can be done while lying on your stomach.

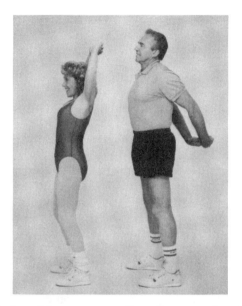

Overhead shoulder press and underarm shoulder press.

Underarm shoulder press. Stand with your feet shoulder-width apart knees relaxed, chest up and shoulders back. Grasp your hands behind your back, bend the elbows and gently push upward until you experience mild tension. Do not bend at the waist or round the shoulders. This exercise can be done while lying on your stomach.

Lower Back

Purpose: To relieve the tightness that results from the continual contraction of these muscles during standing and walking. Tightness in these muscles can lead to low back pain.

Exercises: *Standing back curl.* Stand with your feet shoulder-width apart and knees relaxed. Grasp your hands in front of your shoulders, tuck your chin on your chest, and round out your shoulders and back.

Both knees to chest. Lie flat on your back, head on the floor. Pull knees up toward your chest.

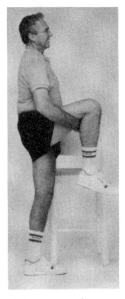

Knee to chest.

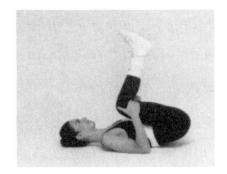

Both knees to chest.

Front of Hips

Purpose: To stretch the hip flexors, which are tightened by frequent and prolonged sitting. This tightness can produce a sway-back posture and lead to low back pain.

Exercises: *Standing hip stretch.* Stand with one foot in front of the other, chest up and shoulders back. Slowly flatten your lower back by pushing your buttocks forward until you feel mild tightness in front of the hip region of your rear leg. Do not lean back or arch the back.

Lunging hip stretch. Assume the lunge position shown in the photograph. Be sure that the front knee is directly over the heel of the foot and not over the toe of the foot. The other knee should be placed on the floor. Support your weight by placing both hands on the floor. Gently flatten your lower back by pushing your buttocks forward until you feel mild tightness in front of the hip region of your *rear* leg. Do not arch the back.

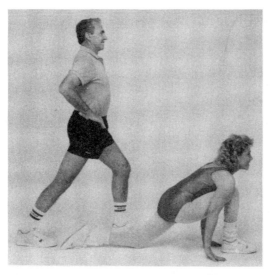

Standing hip stretch and lunging hip stretch.

Front of Thighs

Purpose: To stretch these tight muscles, which often become tight from walking and stair climbing.

Exercises: *Quadriceps stretch.* In a standing position support yourself on a wall or chair. Grasp the outside of the ankle with your hand (same side hand as foot). Gently pull the foot toward your buttocks. Keep the knee pointing straight down. This exercise can be done lying on your stomach. If you cannot reach your foot with your hand, loop a towel around your ankle and gently pull on the towel. *Do not do this exercise if it hurts your knees.*

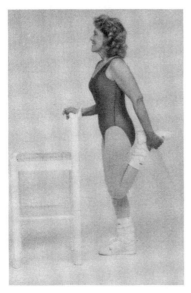
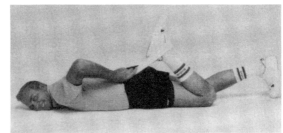

Back of Thighs   **Quadriceps stretches.**

Purpose: These muscles can become tight from sitting with the knees bent, especially when the low back is unsupported in poorly designed chairs and car seats.

Exercises: *Standing hamstring stretch.* Stand with one foot in front of the other. Gently push your buttocks backward until you experience mild tightness on the back of the thigh of your *front* leg. This stretch becomes a little more effective if you place the forward heel on a raised surface.

Lying straight-legged hamstring stretch. Lie flat on your back, head and shoulders down on the floor. Bend one knee to the chest and extend the other leg straight upward. Place your hands behind the thigh and slowly pull the extended leg toward your chest. If you cannot reach your leg without lifting your head and shoulders off the floor, either place a towel around your thigh and gently pull on the towel or do the lying bent-knee hamstring stretch, which follows.

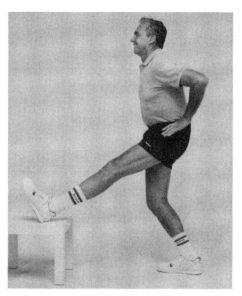

Standing hamstring stretch.

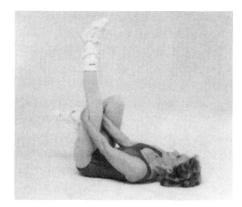

Lying straight-legged hamstring stretch.

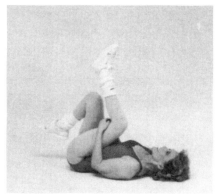

Lying bent-knee hamstring stretch.

Lying bent-knee hamstring stretch. Lie flat on your back, head and shoulders down on the floor. Bend both knees to the chest, grasping one leg behind the thigh. Gently extend the leg to the point of mild tightness while still keeping the knee against the chest.

Calves

Purpose: These muscles are used repeatedly in standing, walking, and climbing stairs, so they become tight, especially in people who regularly wear shoes with raised heels.

Exercises: *Wall press.* Lean against a wall or a sturdy chair, placing one foot behind the other. Keep the rear heel in contact with the floor, both feet pointed forward. Slowly lean forward at the hips until you experience mild tightness in the calf region of the *back* leg. Keep both knees relaxed. To stretch the second muscle of the calf, simply bend the rear knee.

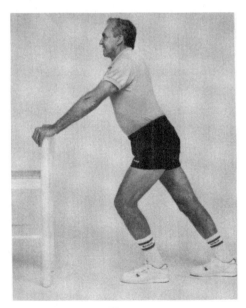

Wall press.

Modified hurdle stretch. Sit on the floor with one leg extended the other knee bent inward. Place a towel around the ball of the foot of the extended leg. Gently pull on the towel. Do not lock the knee of the extended leg. Do not bend over at the waist.

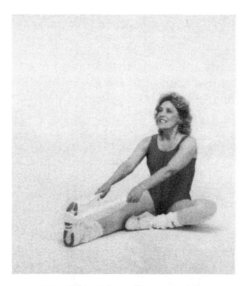

Modified hurdle stretch.

Ten Stretches to Avoid

Over the years, people who exercise have built up a traditional repertoire of calisthenics. Some of these traditional exercises can be effective if they are used for specific purposes, but in many other cases they can actually increase the risk of your becoming injured. There are a number of reasons these potentially harmful exercises are still widely used. Many teachers and coaches do not stay abreast of research, media personalities who have become fitness "experts" without any formal training rely on what they learned back in school, and all of us are continually exposed to television images of successful athletes performing the same warm-up routines that their heroes did a generation ago. Here is a list of stretches you should avoid as much as possible.

1. *Forward leaning while standing*
This position puts uneven and excessive compression on the discs of the lower back, which may result in low back pain.

2. *Forward leaning while twisting*
This exercise not only puts uneven and excessive compression on the discs of the low back, it adds a grinding stress to these discs.

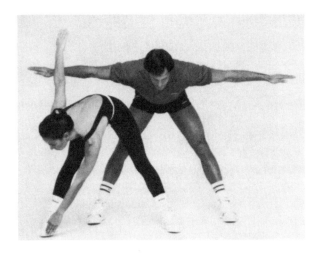

Forward leaning while twisting and standing. (AVOID)

3. *Unsupported standing back arch*
This exercise causes excessive and uneven compression on the discs of the low back.

4. *High kicks*
Many people find it impossible to control the momentum of the leg after it has been swung upward, and this can result in over-stretching of the hamstring muscles on the back of the thighs.

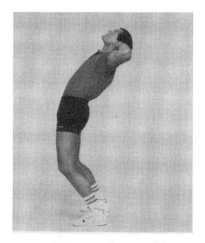

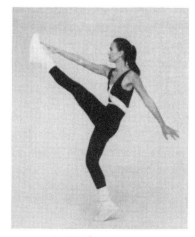

**Unsupported standing
back arch. (AVOID)**

High kicks. (AVOID)

5. *Twisting stretch with feet flat on the ground*
By not allowing the lower body to rotate with the upper body, this exercise places a stressful twisting action on the low back and knee jomts. Simply allowing the rear foot to pivot on the ball of the foot relieves these stresses.

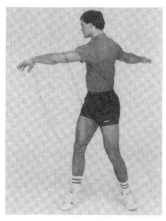

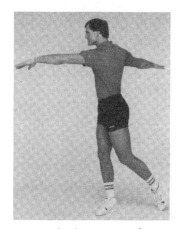

**Twisting stretch.
(AVOID)**

**Twisting stretch.
(CORRECT)**

6. *Sitting hurdle stretch*

This exercise stretches the ligaments on the inside of the rear knee, making the knee joint vulnerable to injury. To modify this position, bend the knee in the opposite direction, bringing the foot to the inside of the knee.

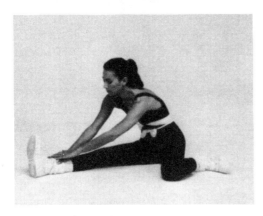

Sitting Hurdle Stretch. (AVOID)   **Sitting Hurdle Stretch. (CORRECT)**

7. *Deep squat*

This exercise can stretch the ligaments of the knees, making them more vulnerable to injury.

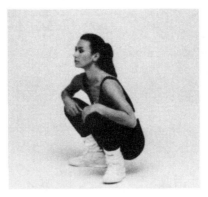

Deep squat. (AVOID)

8. *Kneeling quadricip stretch*

This exercise can stretch the ligaments of the knees, making them more prone to injury.

9. *The Yoga "plow"*

Yoga experts believe that this stretch can be safe and effective when it is performed by a skilled yogi, but for health-related fitness programs the potential risks probably outweigh possible benefits. This body position can put uneven and excessive stress on the intervertebral discs of the neck.

10. *Neck hyperextension*

This also places uneven and excessive stress on the discs of the neck.

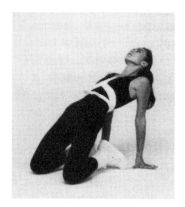 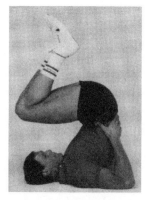 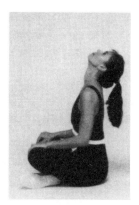

Kneeling quadricep stretch. (AVOID)   **The Yoga "plow." (AVOID)**   **Neck hyperextension. (AVOID)**

FIT TIPS

1. Regular stretching will help you maintain good posture and lessen many common aches and pains.

2. Wear comfortable clothing when you stretch.

3. Move carefully into each stretching position and hold it for at least ten seconds. *Do not bounce.*

4. Stretch to the point of mild tension in the muscle. *Stretching should not hurt.*

5. If the tests in Chapter 3 show that some of your muscles are tight, spend extra time every day stretching those muscles.

6. The most important stretching exercises for most people regardless of their fitness level or the physical activities they perform are: shoulders, page 64; chest, page 64; lower back, page 65; front of hips, page 66; front of thighs, page 67; back of thighs, page 68 and calves, page 70.

7. Warm up your body before you begin to stretch.

8. Stretch *before* and *after* each exercise session.

9. Avoid hazardous exercises such as:

   Standing and bending forward in an unsupported position, page 72.
   Unsupported back arch, page 73.
   High kicks, page 73.
   Trunk twists with your feet stationary, page 73.
   "The hurdler stretch," page 74.
   Deep knee bends, page 74.
   "The plow," page 75.
   Hyperextension of your neck, page 75.

10. If any position or stretch causes you abnormal discomfort, *stop doing it* and consult a fitness expert or a medical professional.

Chapter 6

HOW TO STRENGTHEN YOUR MUSCLES

Muscles that are not used on a regular basis can become progressively smaller and weaker. There is a lot of truth in the old saying "Use it or lose it!"

Although the primary reason for the recent interest in weight training seems to be a concern for physical appearance, the fact that more people are paying attention to the condition of their muscles is an encouraging step toward improving health and fitness, *provided that discriminate strength exercises are being used.* There is no doubt that indiscriminate weight training—that is, randomly performing any old exercises without some logical reasons—can actually do more harm than good.

Take Thomas, for example. He wandered into a weight room having decided that he wanted to improve his strength. He watched what other people were doing and "designed" himself a program that included an exercise that strengthens the calf muscles. Now, Thomas's calf muscles were already tight, and the muscles that tend to counterbalance the calf muscles (situated on the front of the shin) were extremely weak. What he didn't realize was that his indiscriminate weight training program was making his calf muscles stronger and possibly tighter, while the muscles on the front of his shins remained weak. This created a condition known as a *muscle imbalance.* Some time later, Thomas appeared in the office of a sports medicine specialist, complaining of severe pain in his shins, commonly referred to as shin splints. The physician attributed Thomas's shin pain to his muscle imbalance, which had adversely affected Thomas's ability to cope with the repeated pounding on his feet when he walked and ran. Thomas is certainly not unique in his approach to strength training. We can't emphasize enough that each strengthening exercise should be performed with a very specific purpose in mind.

Our lifestyles cause most of us to neglect a number of important muscles, and this can lead to a variety of health problems. But it is usually relatively easy to improve strength to a level where we can maintain good general health and fitness. In fact, of the three components of fitness (strength, flexibility, and cardiovascular endurance), strength training can usually produce the most visible results in the least amount of time.

Training that increases muscle strength also improves muscle-tone. Toned muscles are firm to the touch and have a well-defined or sculptured appearance. A reasonable degree of muscle definition is thought to be attractive in our body-conscious culture. Those people who are interested in the sport of body building obviously have a preference for extreme development and definition of muscles.

In addition to improving muscle tone to enhance appearance, there are a number of more practical reasons for maintaining or improving muscle strength:

1. *Toning and strengthening muscles can also maintain or improve your appearance by ensuring good posture.* If some important muscles are relatively weak compared with others, your posture will tend to slump. This may be due to the activities of daily living, but it may also occur in uninformed people like Thomas who indiscriminately strengthen some of their muscles and neglect equally important ones.

2. *Toning and strengthening muscles enables you to perform daily tasks and recreational activities more efficiently.* Improved strength will make it easier for you to lift and carry heavier loads such as grocery sacks, books,

and growing children, and will help you do tasks that involve pulling and pushing, such as moving furniture and wheeling carts. Improved strength is also essential if you want to improve your speed in aerobic activities such as swimming and running.

3. *Toning and strengthening helps reduce the risk of injury.* Weaker muscles are more easily injured than stronger muscles, and muscle tone helps protect your joints and ligaments so they can withstand stresses they will undergo when you take part in vigorous activity.

4. *Discriminate strengthening of muscles can prevent muscle imbalance.* When a muscle on one side of a joint becomes much stronger than the muscle on the other side of the joint, the risk of injury increases, especially when you take part in strenuous activities. This condition, described earlier, is known as a muscle imbalance. Injuries can occur during sudden and rapid movements produced by the powerful contractions of the stronger muscle. This can stretch the weaker muscle beyond its safe limits so that it becomes torn or pulled. If you make certain that muscles on both sides of a joint are approximately equal in strength this is less likely to occur.

5. *Toning and strengthening increases the mass of muscles, and this in turn increases caloric expenditure.* Muscles burn more calories than any other parts of the body. Therefore, increasing muscle mass will increase caloric expenditure, even at rest. In other words, people with well-developed muscles burn more calories than people who have relatively poor muscle development, even when they are resting.

Janet was a promising young sprinter who had done extremely well in high school track meets. During her second month in college, she exploded out of the starting blocks at the start of a 100-meter training run. After only a few strides she came to an abrupt halt and grabbed the back of her thigh. In excruciating pain, she was taken to the training room. The team physician found that Janet had suffered a severely torn hamstring muscle. After performing some strength tests, the physician concluded that Janet's quadricep muscles (on the front of the thigh) were much stronger than her hamstrings (on the back of the thigh). After her recovery period, Janet modified her training program to include more strength training for her hamstring muscles, and they are now comparable in strength to her quadriceps. She has been injury-free ever since.

Another way muscle imbalance can cause problems is that the muscle tone on either side of any joint has a "teeter-totter" effect on the joint. To understand this, recall the case of Thomas, the weight lifter. The continuous tension in Thomas's strong calf muscles was much greater than the tension in the muscles on the front of his shins. This tended to pivot his feet around his ankle joints and forced them into an extended position in which his toes were lower than his heels when he was resting. Over time, this allowed the stronger calf muscles to become tighter and the weaker shin muscles to become stretched. Eventually, this affected his ability to lower his heels to the ground without putting a great deal of stress on his body. This affected his whole posture.

Another common muscle imbalance occurs in people whose hip flexor muscles (groin muscles) are much tighter than their abdominal muscles (resulting in a swayback posture and protruding abdomen). You may have also seen other examples of muscle imbalances in weight lifters who have spent more time strengthening their biceps and chest muscles than they have spent strengthening the muscles that extend the elbow joints and the muscles that pull the shoulder blades together. Without equal attention to the opposing muscle groups, it is difficult or even impossible to fully straighten the elbow joints, and the rotation of the shoulder joints caused by the tight chest muscles causes the hairy (back) sides of the hands to face in a forward direction when they are walking.

Common Toning and Strengthening Myths

The repertoire of calisthenics that is part of traditional exercise programs is accompanied by a number of deeply ingrained misconceptions about toning and strengthening. In some cases these misconceptions persist because educators have not succeeded in providing alternative information, but in others the situation reminds us of the remarks of the president of a large company that manufactures cosmetics. He said that his factory produces cosmetics, but the stores they supply sell "hope." In much the same way, the fantasies of youth may be more appealing than the straightforward truths about strengthening and toning. These are the seven most common myths:

1. *Myth:* Doing many repetitions of an exercise will remove fat from the area being worked on.

Fact: If this sounds correct to you, you are one of a majority that still believes in "spot reducing." The common belief is that if you do hundreds of arm circles and sit-ups, you will burn fat from your upper arms and abdomen and you will become thinner in those areas. Nothing could be further from the truth! If spot reducing worked, people who sawed logs would have thin arms and people who chewed gum would have thin jaws. To further illustrate our point, Lorna met a young woman who was attempting to break the record for the number of continuous sit-ups, as listed in The *Guinness Book of World Records.* She came to Lorna complaining of excess fat in her abdominal region in spite of the fact that she was averaging over 1,000 situps a day!

Let's dispel the myth of spot reducing once and for all. When you perform short bursts of very vigorous activity, your body burns mostly carbohydrates. When you exercise moderately for longer periods of time, your body primarily uses its slow-burning fuel, which is fat. When you burn fat, your body continuously removes it in small quantities from *all* the many fat storage areas in different parts of your body. You *cannot* selectively remove fat from any one area of your choice.

The reverse is also true. You can't select where your body stores your excess fat. If your caloric intake exceeds the rate at which you use calories through activity, you will accumulate fat. This will be deposited in all available storage areas. Some people store a greater portion of their fat in specific areas of the body, such as the thighs or abdomen; others have fat distributed more evenly all over their bodies. The unique way in which your fat reserves are distributed, known as *fat patterning,* is determined by heredity. Forget the fantasy that you can sweat off the unwanted bulges with rubber suits, ignore the claims that you can beat, roll, or cream them off, and most of all, forget the myth that you can selectively spot reduce them away.

2. *Myth:* Muscle turns into fat when you stop exercising, and fat turns into muscle when you start exercising.

Fact: Muscle and fat are two entirely different tissues; you can't change one into the other. Think about it. You can't change skin into bone or muscle into brain tissue, so why should you be able to turn muscle into fat? Strength training will improve the tone of your muscles but will have little effect on the fat within and surrounding your muscles. Sustained activities will tend to burn fat. The good news, however, is that the combined effect of weight loss and improved tone may give the appearance of fat turning into muscle.

3. *Myth:* "Going for the burn" is the best way to tone and strengthen muscles.

Fact: This is one of the silliest pieces of advice ever given in exercise classes. For many years, endless repetitions of exercises such as arm circles and leg lifts were mistakenly prescribed for the unobtainable goal of spot reducing. Now these same boring, uncomfortable, and pointless exercises are being indiscriminately used in the vain hope of strengthening muscles by "going for the burn." As one eminent sport scientist remarked: "Until the time comes when there is an Olympic event that requires you to do more arm circles than anyone else, there is absolutely nothing to be gained from hours of flapping your arms."

Scientific research has shown that you can't significantly improve the strength of a muscle unless you use progressively heavier loads with a limited number of repetitions. Excessive repetitions with light loads simply fatigue the muscle and bring on a burning sensation, which signals a buildup of waste products and a lack of oxygen in the muscle tissue. Rather than significantly strengthening the muscle, you are training that muscle to be able to perform many repetitions before the onset of fatigue—and to what practical end, since we rarel need to flap our legs and arms in our daily lives? Although some people who are just starting a strength training program may only be able to work with the low resistance provided by the weight of the arms and legs, they will soon need to progress to light weights or elastic resistance (such as rubber bands) if they wish to continue to make significant improvements in strength. If greater strength is needed, it will be necessary to move on to weight training equipment such as barbells and the kind of strength training machines available in gyms and health clubs.

4. *Myth:* Strength training can improve aerobic fitness.

Fact: Strength training does not usually stimulate the heart and lungs in ways that will produce beneficial changes. An activity is classified as aerobic if it uses many of the large muscles to maintain the heart rate at a training level for a continuous period of time. Usually strength training involves intense activity in only a few muscles for a short period of time while all other muscles are being rested.

Some enterprising people have tried to combine weight training with aerobic activity by moving quickly from one weight training exercise to another in an attempt to maintain an elevated heart rate. This technique, known as aerobic circuit training, can add some variety to your exercise program, but even for experienced people this kind of training may be a compromise that does not allow you to meet either your strength or aerobic goals as effectively as possible. If you enjoy this type of training, remember that each exercise involved in a circuit should be done for a reason and that each discriminate exercise should be performed in precisely the way it was designed. This is especially important as you begin to become fatigued.

5. *Myth:* Women who lift weights will develop bulging muscles.

Fact: This is one of the biggest misconceptions facing women. The hormone testosterone controls muscle bulk, and because women have significantly less quantities of this hormone than men, they are highly unlikely to develop bulging muscles. In fact, the American College of Sports Medicine (ACSM) now recommends that all adults should take part in some form of strength training. The average woman who takes up weight training as part of a general fitness program will develop a smoother, more sculptured look than men. You may have seen professional female body builders who have large, bulging muscles, but this is often accomplished with the use of synthetic hormones, which are widely condemned by the medical profession.

6. *Myth:* People who lift weights always lose their flexibility.

Fact: This is true only if they do not stretch regularly. Weight training can tighten muscles, but you can compensate by stretching each affected muscle before and after strength training. Some weight training equipment is designed to allow you to move your joints through their full range of motion. This feature will help prevent muscle tightness.

7. *Myth:* Strong people are strong in all of the major muscles of their bodies.

Fact: Just because someone can lift a heavy weight over his head does not mean he has strong muscles throughout his body. In fact, we have found that many apparently strong individuals actually have weak abdominal muscles. Strength is specific to each muscle in the body. Sometimes even elite Olympic athletes have had unexpected weaknesses in specific muscles, and when they have strengthened them, they have shown dramatic improvements in performance.

Dos and Don'ts of Strengthening and Toning

1. DO wear comfortable clothing that does not restrict your movements.

2. DO warm-up before beginning strengthening and toning exercises. This means nothing more than walking or jogging in place while swinging your arms. The warm-up does not have to be strenuous enough to make you perspire. Mild exercise such as this pre-

pares your body by raising the temperature of the muscles and lubricating the joints.

3. DO stretch all the major muscles you plan to strengthen. Strength training tightens the muscles, so stretching should be considered as much a part of strength training as your shoes are a part of your running or walking program.

4. DO perform strength exercises slowly and precisely. One of the you most common mistakes in strength training is to become more concerned with the *quantity* of training (how much weight we lift or how many repetitions we perform) than with the *quality* of training (how effectively we train). The person who emphasizes quantity often changes the correct position of the body in an unconscious attempt to make the exercise easier. This practice actually strengthens muscles other than the ones intended. Another common fault is swinging or "throwing" body parts or weights instead of moving them slowly and with careful control. For example, if you throw your head and elbows forward when you do curl-ups, the muscles of the arms and neck may actually be doing most of the work. Your abdominal muscles will be getting very little benefit from the exercise. Even if you can do only a few repetitions correctly, you will have a better chance of meeting your exercise goals than if you rapidly perform the same exercises incorrectly.

5. DO perform strength exercises in sets and repetitions. Eight to 12 continuous repetitions of the same exercise are recommended for general fitness programs. This means that your muscles should be fatigued when you have completed 8 to 12 consecutive repetitions. The 8 to 12 repetitions make one set. In order that the muscle can partially recover before it is worked again, it is recommended that you rest the muscle being exercised at least five minutes between sets. A total of two to three sets is often recommended for general fitness programs, but recent research has shown that most of the gain in strength is produced by the first set. In other words, additional strength can be gained from performing a second or third set, but strength training appears to be governed by a law of diminishing returns. If you want progressively great gains in strength, you must work progressively longer and harder to

achieve them. To use your time efficiently, it is best to complete one set of exercises for each of the muscles you are trying to strengthen before performing a second set for any one muscle. For example, if you begin with an exercise for your abdominal by the time you have finished working various muscles of your arms, legs, and back, your abdominals will have rested for at least five minutes, so you can begin a second set of exercises for these same muscles without interrupting your training.

6. DO use the appropriate amount of resistance. In any kind of strength training, the force your muscles must overcome is known as resistance. Resistance can be the weight of parts of your body or weights held in your hands or attached to your body. Or the resistance can be supplied by rubber bands, elastic tubing, springs, hydraulic valves, or a number of other high-tech machines. The important thing to remember is that your muscles cannot tell the difference. Any form of resistance that will allow you to use the range of motion you need and safely provide the necessary force is appropriate for strength training. Remember that you should select the amount of weight that will produce muscle fatigue when you complete 8 to 12 continuous repetitions of the exercise.

As a muscle adapts to the resistance you are using, it needs to be further challenged with progressively greater resistance-if you want to continue to increase the tone and strength of the muscle. As a rule, when you can complete with ease two or three sets of 12 repetitions of light weights, you should gradually and over time increase the resistance, until you are able to perform just 6 repetitions in the third set. Remember that simply increasing the number of repetitions will develop muscular *endurance* rather than significantly strengthening and toning your muscles.

7. DO exhale (breathe out) on the part of the exercise that requires the most effort. For example, as you do a sit-up, you should exhale as the muscles are contracting on the way up, and inhale as you roll back down. Breathe on every repetition. *Never* hold your breath, as this can cause a sudden increase in blood pressure.

8. DO give muscles that have been exercised a day of rest between strength training sessions. You may either do your complete strength training program on alternate days or train your upper

body muscles one day and your lower body muscles the next. Strength training 2 or 3 times a week will produce adequate strength gains for people who are primarily interested in heath-related aspects of fitness.

9. DON'T do strength training without your doctor's approval if you have high blood pressure. Strength training raises blood pressure, especially if you do isometric contractions pulling or pushing against immovable resistance so that your muscles do not lengthen and shorten. For example, this could be a problem for people whose blood pressure is already dangerously high.

10. DON'T do any strength or toning exercise that causes unusual pain or discomfort. Remember that pain is your body's way of telling you something is wrong. Consult a medical expert.

Strength and Toning Exercises

Your body has several hundred different muscles, and many different exercises can be used to strengthen each of them. The exercises we've selected are intended to improve or maintain your body alignment and reduce the risk of injury when you perform vigorous activities. Should you want to become more efficient in a specific sport, you will need to concentrate on the muscles most utilized in the sport. For example, some tennis coaches recommend strength exer cises for the forearm. Swimmers can benefit from strength exercises for the muscles of the back and chest that forcefully pull the arms through the water.

With each of the following strength exercises, we will identify the area of the body to be strengthened and toned, explain the importance of working these particular muscles, and offer you a selection of exercises that accomplish the desired results. The suggested strength exercises can be done inexpensively and at home, using light weights or parts of your body as resistance. When you are doing an exercise for the first time, begin by using the weight of your body to provide the initial resistance. Do as many repetitions as you can up to a maximum of 12. Remember that this first set will produce the greatest strength gain. If you wish to gain additional strength, you should complete all your exercises, then repeat the sequence one to two more times if you can. When you can easily do one, two, or three sets of 12 repetitions, you will need to increase the resistance by using light weights. You can even use resistance provided by an other person. Gradually increase the amount of resistance over a period of weeks until you are satisfied with the results, at which time you can maintain your strength by staying with the same level of resistance. If at any time you feel pain, stop doing that particular exercise and consult a medical expert.

Upper Back

Purpose: Your chest muscles can easily become tight from doing everyday tasks such as driving, reading, eating—all of which require your arms to be pulled in front of you. Lazy posture while sitting and standing can also contribute to this problem. These activities, on the other hand, require very little work from the muscles that pull the shoulders back. The result is a muscle imbalance between the relatively stronger chest muscles and the weaker upper back muscles, which is manifested by an unattractive round-shouldered posture.

Exercise: *Arm lifts.* Lie on your stomach on a bench or the floor. Stretch your arms out to the sides. Gently raise your arms as far as you can, and squeeze your shoulder blades together. Then slowly lower your arms back to the floor. Do not fling the arms. Keep your head and shoulders on the floor at all times. Do not lock the elbows.

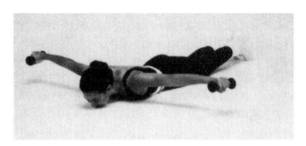

Arm lifts.

Abdominals

Purpose: Because the low back muscles are used continually throughout the day during bending and lifting, and also assist with maintaining an upright posture, they're relatively strong in most active people. Similarly, the groin muscles which flex the hip joints are frequently used during brisk walking and climbing stairs and hills. Most daily activities, however, require very little work from the abdominals. This extremely important group of muscles works in opposition to the low back muscles and hip flexors. This creates a muscle imbalance that often results in low back pain. Most medical experts agree that the combination of weak abdominals and tight hip flexors is one of the major causes of chronic low back pain. Another contributing factor appears to be significant weakness of the muscles that extend the low back region of the spine. Chronic low back pain may affect as many as 80 per cent of all adult Americans. The cost of this widespread complaint in terms of medical treatment and lost productivity has been estimated at a staggering $10 billion to $20 billion each year. A discriminate exercise program could do much to save this money and, more important, greatly reduce suffering.

Exercises: *Pelvic tilt.* This relatively gentle abdominal exercise is particularly suitable for deconditioned people. Stand with your feet shoulder-width apart, knees relaxed, chest up and shoulders back. Slowly flatten your back by pushing your buttocks forward (this is a very small movement). Then return to the starting position. This exercise can be done standing, on your hands and knees, or on your back with the knees bent and the feet flat.

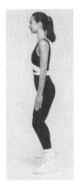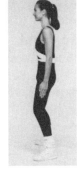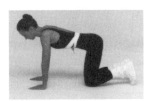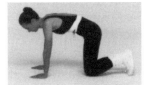

Pelvic tilt.

89

Reverse curl. Lie flat on your back with your knees pulled up to your chest, arms resting comfortably above your head. Contract or squeeze your abdominal muscles until your buttocks move toward your chest. Do not swing the legs. Return to starting position. Again, this will be a very small movement.

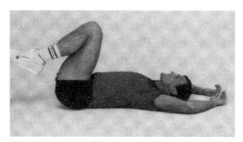 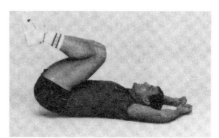

Reverse curl.

Curl-up. Lie on your back, feet in the air or supported on a chair. Clasp your hands behind your head. Press your lower back to the floor. Without pressing the hands against the head or swinging the elbows, slowly curl up, raising the shoulders and upper back off the floor. Slowly curl back down again, this time taking the weight of your head in your hands. Do not allow your lower back to come off the floor. If you have diffficulty raising your shoulders off the floor, place your arms across your chest. (While this is easier on your abdominals, you may find your neck muscles getting tired when unsupported.)

Some respected experts believe that reverse curls and curl-up exercises for the abdominal muscles have some shortcomings. They believe that, for functional reasons, we should train the abdominals to work while the low back is arched in the same gentle curvature that we adopt when we stand upright. Pelvic tilts will allow you to find that position, but conventional reverse curls and curl-ups use a flat position of the low back.

If your abdominals are already fairly strong, and you do not suffer from low back pain, you may be ready to try a more advanced form of curl-up. This involves supporting your low back with a small, soft pad such as a baby pillow or rolled hand towel. This will allow you to begin the exercise in the functional range of movement where the low back is slightly arched. However, the flat backed position described above is less stressful if you are not yet in good shape.

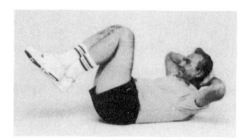

Curl-up.

Front of the Shins

Purpose: The calf muscles are used continually in many everyday activities, but little is required from the muscles on the front of the shins. This muscle imbalance can cause painful conditions such as shin splints and calf pain.

Exercises: *Toe tapping.* Stand with your feet shoulder-width apart, knees relaxed, chest up and shoulders back. Place most of your weight on one foot. Raise the toes of the other foot as high as you can while keeping the same heel on the floor. Bring the toes back down to the floor. Continue tapping motion.

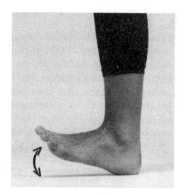

Toe tapping.

Ankle flexing. Sit on the floor with your legs extended, placing your hands behind you for support. Have a partner grasp the top of your foot to resist your movement. Slowly pull the foot toward the knee, while your partner provides just enough resistance to make you work hard. Then continue to contract the same muscles, but allow your partner to slowly extend your ankle joint back to the starting position. Alternatively, you can place an ankle weight around the middle of your foot and then raise and lower your toes while sitting in a chair.

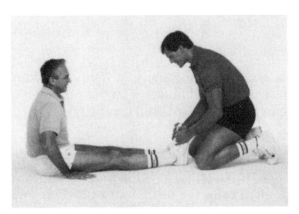 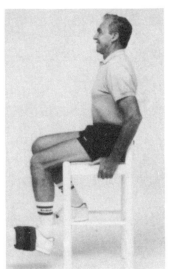

Ankle flexing.

Arches of the Feet

Purpose: The arches are an important part of the body's natural shock-absorbing mechanism. Unfortunately, many people are either born with flat feet or develop them after years of poor health habits. If you have flat feet, you may be mechanically susceptible

92

to painful conditions in the feet and knees. You can maintain the arch mechanism of the foot by strengthening small muscles in the foot and some of the larger muscles in the lower leg.

Exercises: *Toe curls.* Sit or stand with your feet shoulder-width apart, knees relaxed, chest up and shoulders back. Squeeze your toes down toward your heels. Feel your arch rise up off the floor. This exercise can also be done while sitting. For variation, try rolling up a towel with your toes.

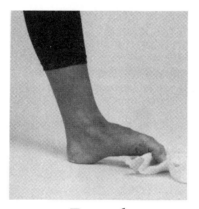

Toe curls.

Ankles

Purpose: Sprains on the outer side of the ankle are relatively common among active people. These injuries can be prevented by strengthening the muscles that tend to keep the sole of the foot flat against the floor.

Exercise: *Ankle rolling.* Place a weight around the middle of your foot. Lie on your side on the floor. Bend the bottom leg slightly for support. You may prop yourself up on one elbow, or support your head in your hand, or extend your arm out while resting your head on it (whichever is most comfortable). Press the outside of the foot upward. Return to your starting position.

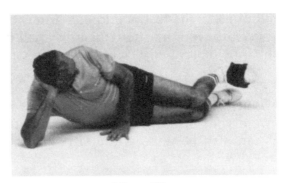

Ankle rolling.

Three Strength Exercises to Avoid

Few people are aware that some popular exercises actually increase the risk of injury. As a result, we often see them used in exercise routines and prominently featured in books and magazines. Remember that as a discriminate exerciser, you do every exercise for a specific purpose and choose exercises which will serve that purpose as safely as possible. So let's discuss the problems associated with performing some potentially dangerous exercises and offer you safer alternatives.

1. *Bending forward in a standing position*
Classical dancers have utilized this position for many, many years, but it is widely agreed that in the absence of good instruction and careful supervision, there is a tendency for most people to flex forward from the lower back, rather than from the hip joints. Strength exercises performed in this position can place uneven compression on the discs of the spine and excessive tension on the ligaments of the low back. Any exercise done in this position is particularly hazardous to anyone with low back pain especially if the stress on the back is increased through the use of hand weights. For safer alternatives, try similar exercises that are done while lying face down on a bench or the floor.

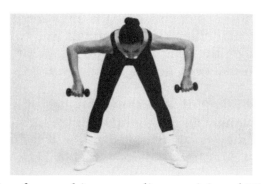

Bending forward in a standing position. (AVOID)

2. *Abdominal exercises with straight legs*

Straight leg sit-ups, V sit-ups, and leg raises are supposed to strengthen the abdominal muscles. However, it is likely that only a few individuals who have superior all-around strength and exceptional control can perform these exercises safely and effectively. For the vast majority of the population, these same exercises performed incorrectly, actually strengthen the muscles that flex the hip joints more effectively than they strengthen the abdominal muscles—so their intended purpose is lost. Even worse, one of the hip flexor muscles (the psoas) tends to pull the low back into a severely curved position when these exercises are done with the legs straight. Exercises done this way can create muscle imbalance between the hip flexors and the abdominals.

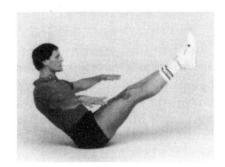
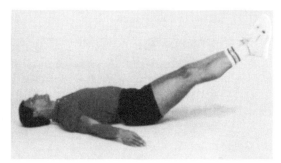

Abdominal exercises with straight legs. (AVOID)

Bent knee curl-ups or reverse curls are a safer and more effective way of strengthening the abdominals (see pages 90–91). This position will keep the back flat on the floor and ensure that you work the abdominals and not the hip flexors.

3. *Arched back while lifting weights*

Hyperextending your back while you are lifting weights places excessive and uneven compression on the discs of the low back. Support your back against the back of a chair or a wall to prevent this problem.

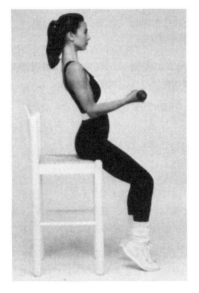
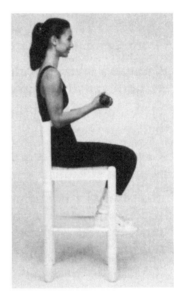

(AVOID)   (CORRECT)

FIT TIPS

1. Strength exercises can help you maintain good posture and body mechanics and lessen many common aches and pains.

2. In order to improve strength, your muscles must work against adequate resistance.

3. Choose a level of resistance that will *just* allow you to perform one, two, or three sets of 8 to 12 repetitions.

4. Muscles should be fatigued when you have completed 8 to 12 repetitions, so give each muscle group at least 5 minutes of rest between sets.

5. Give your muscles a day of rest between strength training sessions.

6. As soon as you can just do three sets of 12 repetitions, you can improve muscle strength by making gradual increases in the resistance.

7. When your body has adapted to the stresses of progressive resistance training, you can continue to improve your strength by using even greater resistance.

8. Do abdominal and upper back strength exercises at least three times a week on alternate days. This will help you avoid pains in your lower back and neck.

9. If you walk, jog, or do aerobics, strengthen the muscles of your shins (page 91) and the sides of your ankle joints (page 93) in order to avoid injuries.

10. Avoid potentially dangerous exercises that involve: Standing and bending over at the waist, page 95. Hyperextending your knees, page 95, your back, page 95. Straight legged sit-ups and leg lifts, page 95.

11. If any body position or exercise causes unusual pain, *stop doing it* and consult a fitness expert or a medical professional.

Chapter 7

HOW TO CREATE YOUR OWN PRE-AEROBIC PROGRAM

Tony was a star on his high school football and baseball teams. During his 5 years in college, he managed to maintain a B average in the School of Business and helped take the football team to a bowl game. After college, for the next 11 years, he found the time to work hard and become the youngest vice-president in his company. He found the time to make some wise investments, and he found the time to become a caring husband and a proud father. Unfortunately, he never seemed to find the time to exercise regularly.

Tony had finally agreed with his wife that it was time for both of them to get back in shape. They had set off jogging together at a leisurely pace, but when Tony remembered how easy it used to be, he decided to sprint the last 50 yards to their front gate. Suddenly, something snapped in his left knee.

Gavin was a "weekend warrior." Monday through Friday he drove his car to the plant, sat in front of a control console for almost eight hours, and then drove home to eat and watch TV. On Saturdays he drove his kids to the pool, the gym, or the baseball field and his wife to the shopping mall. He usually slept late on

Sunday morning. Every Sunday afternoon Gavin played a tough game of basketball.

In the first few minutes of a game Gavin went up for a jump shot from outside of the key. Suddenly, there was a searing pain in his shoulder joint. This was the fourth injury he had had this year. He just couldn't believe his bad luck.

Well-intentioned people often throw themselves into sport and fitness activities with great enthusiasm, believing they can perform just as well as they did before they became inactive. But many of them get hurt and are forced back into inactivity until they recover or until their enthusiasm once more exceeds their better judgment.

The Causes and Prevention of Training Injuries

Research has given us clues to the causes of injuries (like those suffered by Tony and Gavin) and it has also given us insight into how we can stay healthy and active. Exercise physiologists have found that during long periods of inactivity, our bones become gradually less dense-and therefore more brittle and more easily damaged. This process occurs no matter how physically fit a person may have been before inactivity. For example, NASA scientists have found that the bones of superbly fit astronauts become less dense during extended space flights. Bone density changes can also result from a combination of inactivity and a diet low in calcium. This can lead to osteoporosis, or brittle bones, a disease common to elderly women, which often causes bones to break in minor falls.

Ligaments and tendons are more easily stretched or snapped after periods of inactivity. Ligaments are strong bands that attach the bones together and prevent joints from moving into unsafe positions. For example, in healthy individuals the ligaments of the knee will prevent the knee joint from bending either backward or sideways. If these ligaments become damaged, the knee is more vulnerable to injury because it can now exceed the safe limits of its range of motion. Have you ever sprained the same ankle more than once? This is a common problem because once you have permanently stretched the ligaments around the ankle as a result of a severe sprain, your ankle is less stable and more likely to turn over.

Tendons (strong cords that attach muscles to bones) can also be damaged if they are not strong enough to withstand sudden powerful forces during strenuous activities. When Gavin tried a long shot at the basket, he put a great deal of tension on one of the four tendons that hold the arm firmly in the socket of the shoulder joint. Because Gavin's tendon was not resilient enough to withstand the sudden tension, it was severely damaged.

The good news is that the effects of inactivity are reversible for most healthy people. When physical activity is resumed, the ligaments, tendons, and bones slowly become stronger. But it takes at least six to eight weeks of discriminate exercise to produce significant improvements in the strength of these important structures.

Any forms of moderately vigorous activity that repeatedly put moderate tension on the ligaments and tendons will gradually improve their resiliency. For example, a combined program of swimming and walking could improve the resiliency of the ligaments and tendons in both the upper and lower parts of the body.

Research has shown that the most effective way to make beneficial changes in overall bone density is to take part in moderate levels of physical activity such as walking, jogging, dancing, or any other activity in which the feet repeatedly strike the ground. Weight training can also have a similar effect due to the repetitive forces exerted by the muscles on the bones. Nonimpact activities such as swimming and cycling in which the weight of the body is partially supported are less effective, although they can still produce significant improvements in bone density.

By now it should be apparent to you that there is an effective way to avoid the kinds of problems that Tony and Gavin have had. If you have been inactive for some time, you will have to "get in shape to get in shape." You can do just that with a pre-aerobic program.

What Is a Pre-Aerobic Program?

The purpose of a pre-aerobic program is to provide a sensible and gradual progression that will help prepare your muscles, bones, ligaments, and tendons for the inevitable stresses of vigorous exercise. Part of this program consists of stretching and strengthening exercises (Chapter 5 and 6) that were recommended on the basis of your performance on the tests in Chapter 3.

If you are like many Americans who have been inactive for a number of years, the tests in Chapter 3 will probably indicate that your shoulder muscles, chest muscles, hip flexors, back of the thighs, and calf muscles are tight, and your abdominal upper back, and shin muscles are weak. Your posture may also be slumped. Remember that stretching tight muscles can improve body alignment and strengthening weak ones can help stabilize your joints during physical activities.

The other important component of the pre-aerobic program is a carefully controlled progression from gentle activity to moder-

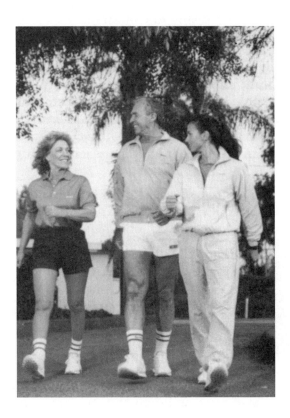

ately strenuous activity. This will allow your body to gradually adapt to the stresses of vigorous exercise over a reasonable period of time. Tony's body was obviously not ready to cope with a stressful activity like sprinting. Gavin's body was never given the chance to adapt to continuous exercise; his occasional games of basketball repeatedly exposed his vulnerable musculoskeletal system to the risk of injury.

Even if you avoid very vigorous activity like sprinting and competitive basketball, there is still a danger of overextending yourself in the early stages of an exercise program. You could be fooled into believing that you are in better shape than you really are—just like Cindy. She began her new exercise program with a one-mile jog every other day. Apart from a little muscle soreness, she did not have any other pains in her bones or joints. The strength of her muscles and the condition of her heart and lungs improved rapidly, and she could soon jog without puffing and panting from the exertion. At this stage she felt extremely invigorated, so she decided to triple her weekly mileage. Soon afterward she began to complain of a sharp pain in her foot. A stress fracture was diagnosed in one of the small bones in the ball of her foot.

On the other hand, there's Marilla. She is a sprightly octogenarian and has been walking briskly and jogging regularly for the past 15 years. So far she has avoided any significant injuries and she intends to keep on moving along for many years to come. It took her 2 years to regain sufficient flexibility in order to begin a running program. Then she cautiously built up her mileage over time, and she avoided any sudden increases in the intensity of her training runs. Undoubtedly, one of the secrets of Marilla's success is her motto, "Consistent moderation is the key to health."

Who Needs a Pre-Aerobic Program?

The pre-aerobic exercise program is designed for people not yet ready to take part in strenuous aerobic activity. Anyone who has been physically inactive for a long period of time is an ideal candidate for this program. The program is also intended for anyone who is significantly overweight or is returning to activity after recuperating from an injury. A shortened version of the program is recommended for active people taking up a new aerobic activity to gradually condition the muscles and joints that will be used.

Pre-Aerobic Activities

You can choose almost any activity or combination of activities you want to prepare yourself for a more vigorous aerobic activity. If you are deliberately preparing yourself for a specific aerobic activity, we suggest you choose at least one pre-aerobic activity that is a modified version of your aerobic activity of interest. For example, if you eventually want to jog, step, slide, skate, or cross-country ski, your best pre-aerobic activity is walking. Gentle movements to music with one foot on the floor at all times would be a good pre-aerobic activity for aerobics; leisurely biking and swimming are appropriate pre-aerobic activities for vigorous biking and swimming. If you are not yet committed to aerobic exercise, we suggest you try a variety of leisurely activities during your pre-aerobic program. You may discover that an activity you had previously not considered is actually more fun than you thought.

You can also include daily activities and recreational outings as part of your pre-aerobic program. Whenever you can, get into the habit of walking a few blocks instead of taking the car or a bus, or walk up stairs in stores and offices rather than relying on elevators and escalators.

There are many different ways of incorporating moderate exercise into *your* program. Perhaps some personal examples will help you think of ways that will suit your unique situation. The two of us have busy teaching and research schedules, and we also have all the commitments that go with raising two active young children. As a result, we sometimes find it difficult to schedule as much *formal exercise* in our daily lives as we would like. So we have learned to incorporate *functional exercise* into our lifestyle. Schedules permitting, Peter rides his bike to the university and Lorna walks the kids to school. On the weekends, we devote at least one day to *fun exercise* in the form of a family outing of hiking, biking, or swimming with the kids.

We have a good friend who has religiously followed an exclusively formal program of running for some years, and she used to tease us about not following her example or "practicing what we preach." Some time ago she spent a vacation with us, and at the end of the week she told us that she was ready to go home and rest for a few days! We compared our activity schedules and found that apart from her one-hour formal exercise session every other day, she actually had a rather sedentary lifestyle. By our estimate, we both probably use about 50 percent more calories every week in our formal-functional-fun exercise program than she does in her formal-only exercise program. The important thing to remember is that your body does not know the difference between physical activity done as a ritual, for fun, or as part of your activities of daily living. As long as the physical activity you do is appropriate for your exercise goals, your body will thrive on it.

One of our strongest recommendations is to mix a variety of activities during the week. This is called cross-training. Triathletes who train in several sports have the right idea. They alternate between running, swimming, and bicycling. Mixing activities not only allows various musculoskeletal structures to rest, thus reducing the risk of injury, it prevents the boredom that often accompanies a single activity. Runners are notorious for complaining about the monotony of the track. A day or two of swimming or biking is an easy solution to the problem.

Guidelines for Increasing Your Pre-Aerobic Activity

Whatever activity you choose, the pace must be leisurely at first, especially if you have been inactive for some time. Use your pre-aerobic activity as a time to socialize with family and friends, enjoy the changing seasons, explore the new neighborhood, or simply take the time to count your blessings. When you begin a new program, the activity should be gentle and comfortable. Initially you should spend only 10 to 15 minutes every second or third day, during which time you should listen to your body. If you feel any unusual discomfort, make adjustments. For example, substituting upright handlebars for curved racing handlebars and changing the height of your seat might make your cycling position more comfortable. Finding shoes that do not chafe your heels will make walking more pleasurable. Using a nose clip to keep water out of sensitive nostrils or finding a pool with warmer water could improve your enjoyment of swimming. Most people who have exercised regularly for many years associate exercise with feeling good. Do not let discomfort spoil your motivation to exercise.

The real key to a successful pre-aerobic program is slow and careful progression. If you have been inactive for a long time, you should take several weeks or even months to gradually increase the amount of time you spend exercising. If you have been exercising once every three days, you can carefully add one more day of exercise during the week, but it is a good idea to make sure that you have a day of rest between each exercise session. In the early stages you should restrict your activity to alternate days, but if you gradually increase the frequency of your exercise, you should mix and match activities so that you can alternate impact activities like walking with nonimpact activities such as swimming and cycling. Finally, when you feel you can handle more activity, you can begin to gradually increase the intensity of the exercise by moving just a little faster or carefully attempting to walk or cycle up progressively steeper hills.

As a further safety precaution, you should avoid making more than one change at any one time. For example, if you have been walking for 20 minutes at a time on flat ground, do not be tempted to walk further if your route will take you up a series of steep hills. If you have been cycling every other day at your own pace, you will probably not be ready to ride for five days each week with a group who cycle much faster than you. Your body may be able to tolerate the extra stress caused by either increasing the total time of exercise or by increasing the severity of the exercise. It is unlikely, however, that you can adapt to greater stresses caused by *both* an increase in time and severity.

Above all, remember that the gradual improvements in the resiliency of your musculoskeletal system are determined by your own unique body. If you enjoy exercising with friends, it is a good idea to find someone who is at about your fitness level so that you will neither be tempted to exceed your present limits nor become bored with the less demanding pace of your companion. Even when exercising with a friend or a group who is at the same fitness level as yourself, be prepared to modify your program in the future if it becomes obvious that you are progressing at a different rate from the rest of the group. If you find that the program is progressing too rapidly, avoid the temptation to follow the crowd when someone suggests another lap around the block, and extra day of training, or a faster pace. On the other hand, if your companions are not progressing as rapidly as you, try to increase the demands of your training in ways that will not make them feel that they have to keep up with you. Remember that all physical activity burns calories. You will burn progressively more calories as you cautiously increase your activity. Although you cannot expect miraculous changes in body weight in a brief period of time, you will be making important changes that will have a cumulative effect on your long-term weight loss goals.

Pre-Aerobic Maintenance Program

You may find that even after six to eight weeks of moderate physical activity, you do not feel ready to begin a more strenuous aerobic program. In fact, you may decide that you are quite content with your new-found activity level. If that's the case, we have some good news. Some of the latest medical research suggests that even moderate amounts of physical activity such as gardening and leisurely walking may reduce the risk of a major heart attack. In fact, many exercise scientists have re-evaluated their position on the type and amount of exercise necessary to stay healthy. Sports medicine experts are now distinguishing between exercise for *health* and exercise for *fitness.* They are recognizing that moderate exercise is beneficial for improving health. It helps people lose excess weight, reduce the risk of coronary disease, maintain adequate flexibility and strength to prevent postural changes, and reduce stress. Individuals who do a great deal of exercise are usually doing so for reasons other than just improving their health. For example, many exercise enthusiasts are interested in improving their personal best marathon times, or training hard to win weight lifting contests or aerobic dance competitions—goals very different from simply improving health.

Moderate levels of exercise help you control your weight by burning calories and by keepng muscles, bones, joints, tendons, and ligaments in good working order. Interestingly enough, a recent study of elderly Americans found that for most of them, musculoskeletal disorders such as arthritis were of much greater concern than heart problems and other fatal diseases. Why? Because musculoskeletal disorders greatly affect one's quality of life on a day-to-day basis. Being physically active and self-sufficient is a great source of pride to many elderly citizens. Crippling musculoskeletal problems inevitably lead to an inability to carry out the simple tasks of everyday living and cause an increased dependency on others. Unfortunately, some people have a genetic predisposition for musculoskeletal disorders, but undesirable stresses on the joints, caused by years of poor body alignment, can create a number of problems and accelerate the onset of others. A discriminate program of moderate exercise can help prevent poor alignment.

Ironically, many people spend more time and effort in planning for their financial security than they do planning for their physical well-being in their advancing years. In these days of rising health costs, many elderly people are spending an increasingly large proportion of their invested resources on health care. Without a doubt, a lifelong program of moderate exercise can reduce the need for a great deal of health care, and may ultimately be a sound financial investment.

You may find that you enjoy pre-aerobic activities and you may even choose not to progress to aerobic exercise. Although you will miss out on some of the more important cardiovascular benefits associated with aerobic exercise, you will still enjoy many health benefits from participating in pre-aerobic activities. It is also possible that you may be like many people who find that the success of a carefully controlled program of this kind will make you feel good about exercise and yourself, and this kind of success can give you the motivation and confidence to expand your exercise goals and move cautiously on to an aerobic exercise program that is right for you.

FIT TIPS

1. A pre-aerobic program is designed to strengthen the bones, tendons, ligaments, and joints of anyone who has been inactive, recently injured, or is planning to start a new fitness activity. It can also begin the process of long-term, sensible weight loss.

2. A pre-aerobic program consists of six to eight weeks of moderate physical activity, together with stretching and strengthening exercises.

3. Progress gradually. Begin with five to ten minutes of leisurely physical activity. As you feel comfortable with the exercise, increase the time by another five to ten minutes.

4. Because pre-aerobic activity is not intense, you can gradually increase your exercise time to 40 to 60 minutes, provided that you do not feel any aches and pains.

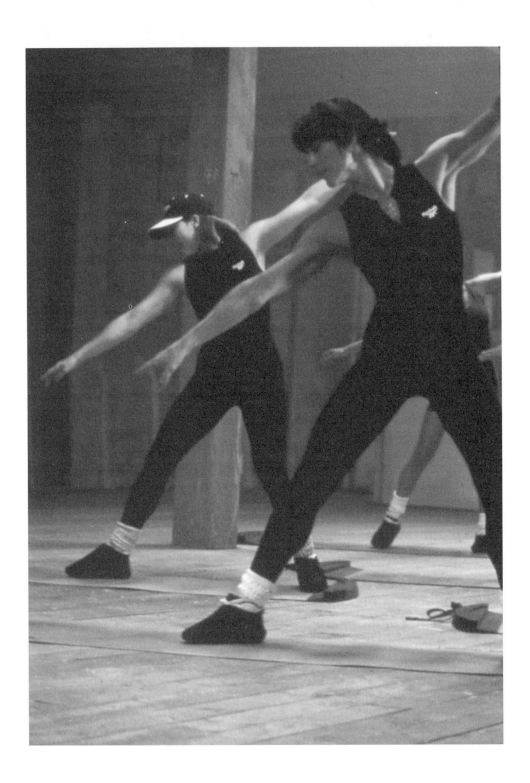

Chapter 8

HOW TO CREATE YOUR OWN AEROBIC PROGRAM

The most exciting development in exercise and physical fitness in recent years has been an increasing awareness that a healthy heart thrives on hard work. The more you make it work, the stronger it becomes. This is hardly surprising, because your heart is actually nothing more than a special type of muscle that contains a series of chambers and valves. Contraction of your heart provides the pumping action that circulates oxygen and nutrients to all parts of your body.

Just like any other muscle, your heart will become stronger when you make it work against resistance. You can increase its workload if you force it to pump larger volumes of blood for an extended period of time. Your heart will automatically do this to meet the needs of the muscles in your arms, legs, and trunk when you use them. The harder each muscle is working, the more blood it will require, the total amount of blood being pumped will increase as you use more and more muscles. Therefore, the best exercise for the heart is *continuous and vigorous exercise* that uses many of your large muscles. This kind of training is known as aerobic exercise.

111

The Benefits of Aerobic Exercise

The improvements in the strength of your heart produced by aerobic training will have a number of other important health benefits:

1. The size of your heart will increase, so it will pump more blood with each heartbeat. Because your heart will be more efficient, it will not have to work as hard and your resting heart rate will go down.

2. The tiny blood vessels that supply your heart with blood will increase in number and in size. Fatty substances that can block the arteries of your heart will also be reduced. These two factors can lessen the likelihood of heart attack.

3. The resistance to the flow of blood through your blood vessels will be reduced, so your blood pressure may go down.

4. Your blood will carry oxygen more efficiently.

5. The same exercise that improves the condition of your heart can also help reduce excess body fat.

6. Many people have found that aerobic activity produces a "natural high" that decreases fatigue and pain. This is attributed to a temporary increase in morphine-like substances in the brain known as endorphins.

7. You will find it easier to perform vigorous activities without feeling uncomfortable, and you will be able to exercise for longer periods of time without getting out of breath.

8. You will recover more quickly after vigorous exercise.

Setting the Limits:
How Much Aerobic Exercise Do You Need?

From a physiological point of view, the more aerobic exercise you do, the better. The benefits listed above will increase as you do more and more aerobic exercise. But research has shown that you must deal with a law of diminishing returns. That is, you must work progressively harder and harder if you want to continue to improve your aerobic fitness. When you first begin a well-designed aerobic program, you will quickly make noticeable improvements. Once your aerobic fitness level is high, making significant changes will become increasingly more difficult. Eventually, you will need a great deal of additional training to gain any noticeable improvements in your aerobic fitness.

Unfortunately, what is good for your heart is not always good for the rest of your body. Any type of sustained aerobic exercise will squeeze, stretch, bend, and twist your bones, joints, ligaments, and tendons. The effect of these stresses will be wear and tear on your body. Your body can miraculously heal many forms of damage. But if the rate of wearing and tearing produced by the exercise is greater than the rate at which your body can heal itself, you *will* become injured. No matter how much you grit your teeth and "suck up the pain," your injury will become progressively worse for as long as you continue to maintain the specific exercise schedule that is causing it.

Aerobic exercise has been called an investment in lifelong health. But it is important to recognize that, just like a financial investment, there is always some risk involved. You should consider and weigh possible risks against potential benefits. In the world of finance, wise investors try to make some kind of compromise that will maximize the potential benefits within the limits of acceptable risks. In the case of aerobic exercise, we can summarize the nature of your investment by examining three broad options.

Option 1: *You can usually expect minimal benefits under conditions of minimal risk.* If you take an extremely conservative approach, you can do little or no aerobic exercise and maintain a low level of cardiovascular health, but the risk of becoming injured is remote. For a number of years before our friend Frank became concerned about his excess weight, his favorite exercise was walking to the refrigerator for another beer during the commercial breaks of Sunday afternoon football games. Frank might have been a good candidate for heart disease, but he never tore a muscle or injured a joint during those sedentary years.

113

Option 2: *To get maximum benefits, you have to be prepared to take maximum risks.* If you do a great deal of aerobic exercise, you stand to gain considerable cardiovascular benefits. But a great deal of exercise will put a great deal of mechanical stress on your bones, muscles, tendons, and ligaments, and your risk of injury will greatly increase.

Option 3: *Giving up some potential benefits can greatly lower the risks.* Your risk of injury decreases as you lower the amount of training you do. In fact, an analysis of running injuries by the National Centers for Disease Control indicated that "the only reasonably well established cause of running injuries is the number of miles run per week." In other words, as mileage goes up, so does the risk of injury. More and more experts are recognizing the long-term advantages of a slightly more conservative approach to training. For example, an eminent coach who trains some of the nation's best middle- and long-distance runners found that athletes who often pushed themselves to their mechanical limits inevitably lost aerobic fitness while they were recovering from their frequent injuries. As a result, those athletes were usually no further ahead of, and were even behind, other top athletes who chose to follow slightly less demanding aerobic training schedules.

The important question is how can you estimate the actual amount of aerobic exercise that is best for *you?* The simple answer is that there is no infallible way to determine the most exercise you can do without getting hurt, just as there is no infallible way of making money on the stock exchange. Many people have consistently made impressive returns on their financial investments, however. In most cases these people have attributed their successes to their *knowledge* of the market. In the same way, you can make discriminate choices about your aerobic exercise program by being knowledgeable about yourself and about the activity or activities available.

Getting Started

If you have not already tried an activity you would like to start, the Aerobic Fitness Assessment in Chapter 3 can help you choose an appropriate entry level for your aerobic exercise program. If you are already taking part in an aerobic activity, you should pay special attention to the guidelines for gradually increasing the amount of exercise you do.

Before you try to make a discriminate choice about the amount of aerobic exercise that is best for you, you should consider guidelines that have been suggested by the most respected professional organization in the field of exercise, at the American College of Sports Medicine. These guidelines are based on hundreds of research studies dealing with aerobic exercise. The guidelines provide recommendations for exercise based on:

1. How often you should exercise.

2. How long you should exercise.

3. How hard you should exercise.

How often should you exercise? In order to improve or maintain good aerobic fitness, you should do aerobic exercise *three* to *five* times each week. In the early stages of your program, however, you should begin with the minimum of *three times each week or less,* so that your musculoskeletal system has a chance to adapt to the new stresses. The best way to do this is to have at least one full day of rest between aerobic exercise sessions. Of course, you can still work on your flexibility and strength on those days when you are resting from aerobic exercise. As your fitness improves, you can eventually progress to the point where you are doing aerobic exercise seven times every two weeks, and still including a day of rest between sessions (Monday, Wednesday, Friday, and Sunday one week, Tuesday, Thursday, and Saturday the following week.)

Many of the exercise enthusiasts we have talked with have told us that a maximum of three or four aerobic sessions each week has allowed them to meet their fitness goals. If you find that this is also true of you, you will be able to give your body a reasonable amount of time to repair itself from wear and tear between exercise sessions. But if your exercise goals involve greater improvements in your aerobic fitness than you can achieve with three or four sessions each week, you will inevitably expose yourself to an increased risk of injury.

We believe this is where cross training (mixing and matching aerobic activities) can help. If you choose to exercise more than four times a week, you can alternate your favorite activity with one or more different aerobic activities that will rest the parts of your body most stressed by your favorite activity. This way you can still give the affected parts of your body a day of rest between exercise sessions. Triathletes, who alternate running with cycling and swimming, seem to be injured less often than runners, who spend the same number of hours in training as the triathletes: good example of the wisdom of mixing and matching aerobic activities.

How long should you exercise? The American College of Sports Medicine guidelines indicate that you can improve or maintain good aerobic fitness by exercising at least *12 minutes* each session. The maximum length of training sessions recommended by the ACSM is *one hour.* If you have been inactive for some time, you should be more concerned about getting used to the aerobic activity than about the immediate aerobic benefits. In this case, we recommend that you not exceed the minimum of 12 minutes in the initial stages of your exercise program. When you feel that you can handle more exercise, you can cautiously increase the length of each training session. Most experts believe that the key to safety is *slow progression* over a period of weeks or months. It takes time for your cardiovascular and musculoskeletal systems to adapt to the new stresses exercise places on them. The longer you exercise in any one session, the greater the stress on your body. Remember, discomfort is a sign that your body is adapting to aerobic exercise, but pain is your body's way of telling you something is wrong. *If it hurts, don't do it!*

The best rate of progression for *you depends on your* unique body. Thus there are no hard and fast rules for deciding how quickly you should increase your training. As a general guide, you should avoid sudden increases in the amount of training that you do. Have you noticed that some top long-distance runners are often injured just before a big race? Many highly trained athletes drive themselves to the limits of their mechanical tolerance when they increase their aerobic training before major competitions. Many physicians who specialize in sports medicine are convinced that a large percentage of the injuries they treat are the result of sudden increases in training.

If you have been inactive for a number of years before you start an exercise program, it would be wise to be especially cautious when you begin to increase the amount of aerobic exercise you do. For example, if you find that a 12-minute session of aerobic exercise is relatively easy, you might decide to increase the duration of each workout rather cautiously by one minute each week. Therefore, it will take 18 weeks to gradually increase your workout from 12 minutes to 30 minutes of continuous exercise. If you increase the duration of each workout by two minutes per week, you would progress to a 30-minute workout in only 9 weeks. On the other hand, if you have been fairly active on a regular basis, you should listen to your body; if you do not feel marked discomfort or pain, you can cautiously increase the length of your exercise sessions at a faster rate. Finally, recent research conducted by Stanford University has indicated that, *for deconditioned people*, three separate 10-minute bouts of exercise in any one day may have the same overall benefits as one single 30-minute session of aerobic exercise. This is good news for deconditioned people, especially for those who find longer bouts of aerobic exercise to be uncomfortable. However, as the fitness level increases, longer sessions of more intense exercise are necessary to produce significant changes in aerobic fitness.

How hard should you exercise? This aspect of exercise is the most difficult to understand, because it is not easy to accurately measure the *intensity* of exercise—that is, how hard you are working. Experienced athletes become extremely good at assessing how hard they are training, but the best guide for most of us is our heart rate. As you work harder and harder, your heart will beat faster and faster to supply blood to your working muscles. The ACSM Guidelines suggest that you can improve or maintain aerobic fitness if you exercise for at least 12 minutes with your heart beating at a minimum of "50% heart rate reserve." This means that your heart rate should be at least halfway between your resting heart rate and your maximum heart rate. Your maximum heart rate is the fastest your heart will beat if you exercise as vigorously as you possibly can, and your heart rate when you wake up after a good night's sleep is your resting heart rate.

Of course, competitive athletes often train much closer to their maximum heart rates, but as we have repeatedly emphasized, you are likely to increase your chances of becoming injured as you work harder and harder. If your exercise goals do not include success in high-level competition, we recommend that you not exercise with your heart rate faster than 75 to 80 percent of the way between your resting heart rate and your maximum heart rate.

Incidentally, the ACSM recommend an upper limit of 90 percent, but they also warn of the possible dangers of working at high exercise intensities. We believe that our recommended upper limit is entirely consistent with the ACSM guidelines for noncompetitors. We should also mention that the ACSM has recently reevaluated the guidelines in light of recent research that seems to indicate we can actually improve or maintain good aerobic fitness with *less* exercise than was previously thought.

The range of heart rates that will produce aerobic benefits is known as the *target heart rate range.* When you are trying to achieve your aerobic exercise goals, you should try to make the most improvements you can within conditions of reasonable safety. You can do this by making sure that your heart rate stays between the upper and lower limits we have suggested. Your *aim* is to exercise so that your heart rate falls within the *target range.* Before you try to find your own target heart rate range, you will need to be able to estimate your resting pulse rate and your exercise heart rate.

Your Resting Pulse Rate

When you wake up each morning, your heart will usually be beating more slowly than at any other time of the day. Place your fingertips on the pulse in your wrist (close to the base of your thumb) and use your watch or bedside clock to count the number of heartbeats in one minute. Or you can use the pulse just to the side of the windpipe in your neck. You will find that the number of beats in a minute will vary a little from day to day; the average value over several days is your resting heart rate. You can use this value as a way of measuring improvements in your aerobic fitness: *Your resting heart rate will go down as your aerobic fitness improves.*

Your Exercise Heart Rate

When you are just beginning an aerobic exercise program, it is important to monitor your heart rate periodically during the exercise session. When you become fitter, taking your pulse at the end of each exercise session will be all that is necessary. With practice, you will become very proficient at quickly estimating your exercise heart rate.

When you took your *resting* pulse rate, you counted the number of beats in one minute. But if you try to take your *exercise* heart rate for a full minute, your heart will begin to slow down when you stop exercising to take your pulse. Exercise physiologists have found that you can get a better estimate of your exercise heart rate if you take it for only ten seconds after you have stopped exercising. Of course, you can easily convert this to the number of beats per minute by multiplying the number of beats in a ten-second period by six.

Your Target Heart Rate Range

You can easily find your target heart rate range in Chart 1.

Step 1: Find the column that is closest to your age.

Step 2: Find the row that corresponds to your resting heart rate.

Step 3: Move one finger down the age column and another finger across the heart rate row to the box where they cross.

The first number in the box is your lowest exercise heart rate for aerobic benefits (50 percent heart rate reserve) The second number is our recommended upper limit for health-related aerobic exercise (75 percent heart rate reserve).

We have tried to make your job easier, however, by giving the values of your target heart rate range in Chart 1 in a ten-second period so that you do not have to do any calculations.

Let's take an example of the way you can use Chart 1. If you are 25 years old, and your resting heart rate is 80 beats per minute, your

119

Chart 1
TARGET HEART RATE ZONES
(Numbers in boxes are pulse counts per ten seconds)

RESTING HEART RATE	AGE						
	15	20	25	30	35	40	45
50	21-28	21-27	20-26	20-26	20-25	19-25	19-24
55	22-28	21-27	21-27	20-26	20-25	20-25	19-24
60	22-28	22-28	21-27	21-26	20-26	20-25	20-24
65	23-28	22-28	22-27	21-26	21-26	20-25	20-24
70	23-29	23-28	22-27	22-27	21-26	21-25	20-25
75	23-29	23-28	23-28	22-27	22-26	21-26	21-25
80	24-29	23-28	23-28	23-27	22-26	22-26	21-25
85	24-29	24-29	23-28	23-27	23-27	22-26	22-25
90	25-29	24-29	24-28	23-28	23-27	23-26	22-26

	50	55	60	65	70	75	80
50	18-23	18-23	18-22	17-21	17-21	16-20	16-20
55	19-24	18-23	18-22	18-22	17-21	17-20	16-20
60	19-24	19-23	18-22	18-22	18-21	17-21	17-20
65	20-24	19-23	19-23	18-22	18-21	18-21	17-20
70	20-24	20-24	20-23	19-22	18-22	18-21	18-20
75	20-25	20-24	20-23	19-22	19-22	18-21	18-21
80	21-25	20-24	20-23	20-23	19-22	19-21	18-21
85	21-25	21-24	20-24	20-23	20-22	19-22	19-21
90	22-25	21-24	21-24	20-23	20-22	20-22	19-21

exercise heart rate range is from 23 to 28 beats in a 10-second count. As we mentioned, this actually represents a range from 138 beats per minute (23 × 6) to 168 beats per minute (28 × 6). If your resting heart rate and age are not included in Chart 1, or if you wish to work more intensely than 75 percent, you can calculate your own target heart rate range using the formula given in Appendix A.

Many people rely exclusively on measuring their heart rate to determine exercise intensity. With practice, however, you may find you will become sufficiently in tune with your body to be able to sense how fast your heart is beating during exercise. This technique, called *perceived exertion,* is particularly useful for skilled exercisers. The best way to improve your accuracy at predicting your exercise heart rate is to try to estimate your heart rate immediately before you actually take your pulse. Then compare your estimate with the heart rate you count. Many people find that their estimates become progressively better over time. When you are sufficiently confident in your ability to use perceived exertion, you may decide to rely exclusively on this technique to estimate exercise intensity.

The perceived exertion technique has another important application. Some people do not have a normal heart rate response to exercise and therefore can't obtain an accurate estimate of exercise intensity from pulse monitoring. Such people include cardiac patients, diabetics, pregnant women, and anyone taking high blood pressure medication that contains beta blockers. If you are in any of these categories, you should seek expert advice from your physician about ways you can use the perceived exertion technique.

We have discussed several techniques for monitoring exercise intensity. But what determines the intensity of your exercise? This varies greatly from activity to activity, but as a general guide, intensity increases as you move faster, or against greater resistance. If you take your exercise heart rate and find that it is too low, you can pick up the pace in running, swimming, and in-line skating, choose faster music or cover more floor space in dance exercise, increase step height or incorporate more powerful moves in step training, and cycle uphill or against headwinds. If your exercise heart rate is too high, you can slow down, cover less space, or reduce the resistance to your movements.

Recovery Heart Rate

As your aerobic fitness improves, your heart rate will return much sooner to its resting level after vigorous exercise. You can

121

use this to measure improvements in your level of fitness. As you get into the habit of checking your exercise heart rate at the end of each exercise session to see whether you have stayed in your target heart rate range, you should also get into the habit of taking your recovery heart rate some time after you have stopped exercising. The exact length of time you wait to take your recovery heart rate is not critical, but anywhere from two to five minutes after exercise works well. The important thing to remember is that the time delay you choose should always be the same. As long as your exercise sessions involve about the same amount of exercise, and if you always take your recovery heart rate at, say, three minutes after you stop exercising, you will be able to measure your progress. Recovery heart rate will fluctuate from session to session, but if you look for a general trend, you should spot a downward change in your recovery heart rate, which indicates improvement in your aerobic fitness.

Warming Up

Before you begin any vigorous physical activity, you should always warm up your body with a few minutes of light exercise and some stretching. Warm-up exercise is *not* meant to be vigorous, and it should not make you breathe heavily. Its purpose is to raise the temperature of your muscles and lubricate your joints so that you can perform comfortably and safely. You can achieve this many different ways. Some track athletes begin by walking while they gently move their arms in large circles. Most cyclists warm up by riding in low gear at an easy pace, and swimmers usually warm up with a few laps of relaxed swimming. You can choose any form of easy activity that is convenient and feels good. There is no hard and fast rule about how long you should spend warming up, but in general it will take longer in cold surroundings. When warming up becomes a habit, you will learn to recognize when your body is ready for you to start stretching. Before beginning vigorous exercise, spend a few minutes stretching the muscles that will be used in your chosen physical activity. This will help you perform the activity safely and efficiently. Once you have completed the stretching, you need to *gradually* increase the intensity of your aerobic activity. Sudden strenuous exercise can cause an insufficient flow of blood to the heart muscle, which in rare cases can actually damage the heart.

Aerobic Activities: Making Discriminate Choices

Remember: Any activity that uses many of the large muscles your body for an extended period of time can be used for aerobic exercise. Running, walking, aerobics, step training, slide training, swimming, cycling, rope jumping, rowing, kyaking, canoeing, and cross-country skiing are all effective forms of aerobic training. Some of these activities are also recognized as competitive sports, and many people like to combine their aerobic training with the excitement of competition. Even though the vast majority of people who walk and do aerobics are primarily interested in fitness, racewalking and aerobics competitions do attract some enthusiasts. For competitive people, the challenge to strive to be the best adds another dimension to the quality of life. "The thrill of victory and the agony of defeat" can be memorable events in our personal growth.

However, we believe that many of the misunderstandings about exercise have arisen from our national obsession with sports competition. Research has shown that one of the characteristics of people who have a high degree of motivation to succeed in competition is that they are prepared to take considerable *risks.* An increased risk of injury is acceptable to many sports competitors who want to increase their chances of victory.

There is no doubt that many people who use sports activities to meet their exercise goals have been affected by role models who are successful competitors in those sports. Competitors will talk about "a short run of four or five miles" or "an easy ten-mile ride." Either of these feats is well beyond the capabilities or needs of many untrained people. In some of the more macho sports, injuries may be regarded as honorable "battle scars," and many ordinary folks whose primary goal is to improve general health are often misled into thinking that injuries are inevitable if they use these sports activities as part of their exercise programs.

If your exercise goals do not include success in competition, you can still make a discriminate choice to use an aerobic sport activity as part of your fitness program. But remember that your exercise goals should dictate how much activity you need to do. Ignore the advice of your competitive friends and ignore the magazines and books that are written for the performer who wants to succeed in competition. *Your* aerobic fitness program should help you meet your exercise goals.

In addition to the popular activities already mentioned, the appeal of aerobic training has also encouraged the development of some ingenious machines that can be used at home or in gyms, clubs, and health spas. Treadmills move the floor surface underneath your feet while you walk or run in place, and many of them can be slanted so that you must in effect walk or run up a continuous incline. Exercise bicycles, rowing machines, slide boards, and cross-country ski simulators can provide exercise similar to outdoor cycling, rowing, skating, and skiing. Minitramps, or rebounders, provide exercise that is similar to trampolining, and other devices allow you to perform movements that resemble stair climbing.

In summary, an exhilarating array of aerobic exercise opportunities is available, and almost everyone should be able to find at least one activity that is available, affordable, effective, and enjoyable. But before you choose an aerobic activity for *your* program, it is important to examine the benefits and risks involved in each one so that you can make your own discriminate choices, rather than choices based on the advice of well-meaning friends and/or common misconceptions .

Running

> *"Birds fly and Ashes swim; running is the purest and most natural thing that human beings can do. When I run, the Free Spirit inside of me takes over and I am a carefree child again."*—P. R. F., London, England

Running, or jogging, as it has become to many exercise enthusiasts, can be done in almost any open space. Apart from a good pair of shoes and a minimum of clothing, there need not be any financial cost. For many people, running is a scheduled part of their lives; certain times are set aside for a regular run. Generally speaking, running falls into the category of formal exercise, but for many it is also fun exercise. Running can be a social time with friends, and if you become bored you can run together in new places. No doubt there has been more said in praise of running than any other exercise activity in the history of mankind. The good news is that *most of what has been said is true. The bad news is that some* of the things that have been done and said have been completely wrong.

Not everyone was born to run! Look around you. Your common sense will convince you that this is true. Some time ago we met Charlotte, a striking example of this simple fact of life. Charlotte had flat feet, she was severely knock-kneed, and she was at least 40 pounds overweight. If she had had the opportunity to take the tests in Chapter 3, it would have become immediately obvious that she should have sought expert advice before deciding to start a jogging program. Don't get us wrong. We have a great deal of admiration for Charlotte. She made a real commitment to improving her health and she did not give up easily.

By the time she visited a sports medicine clinic, she could hardly walk. Both knees were swollen and she had a great deal of pain in one foot. The amazing thing is that she was still committed to exercise. Fortunately for Charlotte, she came under the care of an excellent doctor. After a brief period of inactivity, she began a stretching and strengthening program. Then she enrolled in an Aquarobics class and began exercising to music in chest-deep water. She was also fitted with in-shoe orthotics and has now started to walk regularly with a group of her neighbors. Charlotte has a terrific sense of humor. The last we heard, she was planning to start a group called Jog-aholics Anonymous. She says that anyone who is not cut out for running and who has an overwhelming urge to start to jog should call her, and she will talk them out of it.

Eleanor carries herself with the easy grace that comes with supple joints and good posture. Her hips are narrow and she has striking muscle definition that is evidence of her good muscle tone and relatively low body fat. When she runs she seems to move effortlessly over the ground rather than pounding it with her feet. She runs three or four times a week and has had no serious injuries in the six years she has been running. Eleanor *was* born to run!

Research has shown that running is a superb aerobic activity, but unfortunately, many runners do get hurt. Most commonly injured are the knees, heel cord, shins, the sole of the foot, and the low back. Quite simply, if you have already been injured in one or more of these areas of your body, you should either avoid running or progress cautiously when you start a running program. Many experts agree that the repeated pounding of your feet against the ground or pavement can cause a number of injuries in the feet, shins, knees, and low back, and that those runners who over-pronate are especially suceptible to injuries to the knees and shins. Choosing suitable shoes and running on nonrigid surfaces can cushion impacts to your feet. Motion control can be improved with orthotics and appropriate shoes. On the other hand, excessively soft running surfaces can allow your feet to roll freely inward and create overpronation.

Walking

> *"I would have felt rather silly running at my age; walking feels right for me."*—E. G., Montreal

> *"I used to fight my way through traffic every morning and get to work all stressed out. Now that I walk, I can plan my whole day and get there feeling great."*—P. C., Minneapolis

> *"I love to run, but I had one injury after another. Now that I am walking regularly, I don't get hurt anymore. The funny thing is, I know that I have lost more weight walking than I ever did running."*—N. N., Boston

Walking has rapidly become the most popular exercise activity in the country. According to the National Sporting Goods Manufacturers Association, there were 23.2 million people who walked for exercise in 1987. By 1994, the number had soared to 35.8 million. Walking was by far the most popular choice for females who exercised regularly in 1994, and the number of males who walked regularly was only exceeded by the numbers of males who used free weights on a regular basis. In fact, it is likely that more people are now walking for exercise than were running at the height of the "jogging boom." We see people of all ages walking everywhere—on sidewalks, trails, and even around indoor shopping centers in cold or wet weather. One of the great advantages of walking is that you can use it in any of the three categories of exercise: It can be formal, it can be functional, and it can be fun. If you are a disciplined person who likes to schedule exercise to meet your needs, you can include a brisk walk as a formal part of your program. If you are a busy individual who finds it hard to schedule a regular exercise session into an unpredictable lifestyle, you can use walking as a functional part of your day. That is, you can walk to the grocery store, to your job, or to pick up the kids from school. Finally, walking can be fun if you like to socialize. Unlike many other physical activities, walking will allow you to carry on a conversation comfortably; you can exercise while you plan, reminisce, or just plain gossip with your family and friends. With the ever-increasing numbers of people walking, you can even use walking to make friends.

Walking is less stressful on the musculoskeletal system than running. Scientific measuring devices have shown that the impact force on the heel for most runners is two or three times the weight of the body each time a heel strikes the ground. The same force during walking usually drops to less than one and a half times the weight of the body. These differences are due to the fact that you always have at least one foot supporting the weight of your body while you are walking, but when you run you literally fall downward onto one heel at the end of each stride.

Even though walking is easier on your body than running, it can still cause pain and injuries. The most common problems are fairly trivial things like blisters, which can be prevented by discriminate choices of shoes and socks. It is a good idea to break in new walking shoes by cautiously trying them close to home before you set off on a long hike.

A few walkers have suffered injuries to their feet, ankles, knees, hips, back, and groin. In other words, walking injuries tend to be similar to running injuries, but they occur far less frequently and tend to be less serious. The tests in Chapter 3 should reveal shortcomings that might create problems, and in some extreme cases, especially involving excessive body weight, it is wise to start on flat ground at a leisurely pace.

Aerobics

> *"Dance exercise is my passion, my release, my joy. It lets me get rid of my emotional stresses and be anything I want to be. I can fantasize while I give myself the priceless gift of health."*—Judy Shephard Missett, founder and president of Jazzercise, Inc.

> *"Aerobics saved my life. I was ready to sit down and fade away. Now I can't wait to get to class, and I feel better than I did 20 years ago when I was 52."*—M. L., Los Angeles

Aerobics, which is often called aerobic dance or dance exercise, has been phenomenally popular since it was introduced in 1969. Like any other effective form of exercise, it has undergone many new and exciting innovations, and there is now a wide variety of different styles of exercise to music that are collectively known as aerobics. These include different forms of dance exercise known as high impact and low impact aerobics, as well as aquarobics, step training and slide training.

Dance Exercise

Traditional dance exercise has been more popular with women than with men, but today many programs are attracting men in ever increasing numbers. Dance exercise differs from most other aerobic activities in that it is done in a group setting under the supervision of an instructor. Classes usually meet on a regular basis,

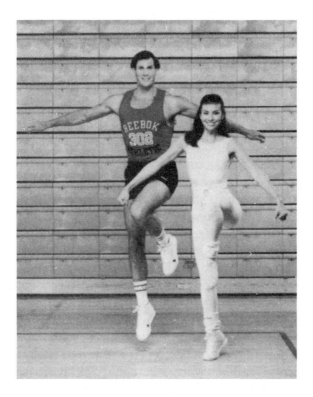

so it is ideal for those people who like regularly scheduled formal exercise. Group participation to the accompaniment of popular music has also made dance exercise fun for millions of enthusiasts. The flattering exercise clothing now available has also helped make this popular activity as much a social event as an effective form of aerobic exercise.

Like any other aerobic exercise, dance exercise can cause injuries. The parts of the body most often affected are the shins, followed by feet, back, ankles, and knees. Most researchers believe these injuries are caused in the same way as injuries suffered by runners. That is, repeated pounding of the feet on the floor can produce stresses that exceed the tolerance limits of the bones, muscles, tendons, and ligaments. Overpronation can also be stressful to the knees and shins.

If you have already suffered injuries to any of the vulnerable regions listed above, you should either choose an activity that is less

129

stressful on your body or try a beginning-level class that meets only two or three times a week. Many experienced instructors now offer low-impact aerobics classes designed to minimize the stresses on your feet, legs, and back.

Aquarobics

Aquarobics classes, conducted in waist-deep or chest-deep swimming pools, are ideal for people who have had a history of injuries or who are obviously overweight. There are a number of advantages to exercising in water. The buoyancy of the water reduces the pounding on your feet, and prevents fast uncontrolled movements that may be stressful to vulnerable joints. This kind of training is being used by some of the world's best athletes when they are injured, but you may remember the fun you had when you were a kid splashing about with your friends in a pool, lake or the ocean. Try it again. It may be the most fun you have had in a long time. If your tests in Chapter 3 indicate flexibility or strength deficiencies, you should begin with a pre-aerobic program that stresses stretching and strengthening exercises for your shortcomings. Refer to Chapters 5 and 6 for specific exercises.

Step Training

Step training, or step aerobics, was conceived by Gin Miller of Holly Springs, Georgia, in 1986. With the assistance of a team of researchers and educators assembled by the Reebok Corporation, the activity has rapidly developed and become immensely popular all over the world. Our own research has shown that step training can be a highly effective form of aerobic exercise, and the injury rate is remarkably low.

Occasional injuries to the knees are probably due to stepping on an excessively high platform, or attempting to twist the body (pirouette) while one foot is firmly planted on the platform. Injuries to the heel cord (Achilles tendonitis) or pain in the sole of the foot (plantar fasciitis) are probably due to poor stepping technique.

That is, stepping too far back from the platform creates a great deal of tension in the heel cord when the heel is lowered towards the floor. Stepping up on to the platform with the heel unsupported over the edge of the platform will place excessive tension on the calf muscles and also on the sole of the foot.

If you wear glasses, and especially if they have bifocal lenses, be cautious when you are step training, as they may restrict your vision when you glance downwards to locate the edge of the platform.

Slide Training

This exciting form of aerobic exercise evolved from a training technique that has been used for many years by successful speed skaters when ice is not available. Continuous contact between at least one of the feet and the slide board creates a "low impact" aerobic workout. With practice, the simpler side-to-side sliding movements can be done by deconditioned people, but the more vigorous moves done at higher cadence provide a very high-intensity workout.

The injury rate appears to be extremely low, but individuals who suffer from low back pain should restrict the amount of time they spend in the "speed skate" or "low profile" position in which the trunk is flexed forward and parallel with the floor. In order to maintain safe and consistent sliding conditions, slide boards should be kept clean. Clean nylon socks should be worn over comfortable, well fitting shoes that provide a stable base of support.

Before you select any music-based aerobic exercise program, give some thought to making a discriminate choice based on the instructor's qualifications. Some classes are offered by self-taught instructors, but awareness is growing that a trustworthy instructor should have training in the scientific aspects of exercise. A number of excellent training programs are now available, and many instructors have become certified by one or more nationally recognized professional associations.

As an alternative to joining a class, many people choose to exercise at home with aerobics videotapes. This may be the only choice if no classes are available in your immediate neighborhood. Many exercise videotapes feature show-business celebrities as role models, and these well-known figures have served as good examples of physical fitness for many people who would otherwise be unwilling to exercise. But many of these celebrity videotapes contain indiscriminate exercises that have caused pain and injuries to people who have tried to do them at home. Exercise programs based solely upon the commercial appeal of celebrities are likely to be no more effective than programs devised by any other individual who has little or no training in medicine or science. Many of the more popular health and fitness magazines regularly review and rate exercise videotapes. These reviews are particularly valuable if the critic is also a fitness expert.

Swimming

> "When I swim, I'm in my own tranquil and weightless world. I can lock out work, worry, and even the kids for a part of every day."—S. B., San Diego

There is some uncertainty about whether swimming or walking is now America's favorite exercise activity, but there is no doubt that swimming has been and will continue to be enormously popular. Unlike running and walking, which provide a great deal of activity for the legs, swimming relies to a great extent on the muscles and joints of the arms and shoulders. It also offers some variety by allowing you to change from one stroke to another whenever you feel like it.

Water supports the weight of your body and it also tends to prevent you from making rapid, uncontrolled movements that can put harmful stresses on your musculoskeletal system. For this reason, swimming is often used in rehabilitation programs for people who are recovering from serious injuries or recent surgery. Swimming is also ideal for many people who have problems with body alignment or who are severely overweight and would probably find many other activities extremely stressful.

Swimming can be included in your exercise program in a formal way if you wish to schedule regular sessions of lap swimming at your local pool, but it can also be fun exercise, especially if you enjoy the outdoors and have access to lakes and the ocean. For some people, a fear of water or sensitivity to water chemicals can discourage them from taking part in this activity which might otherwise be ideally suited to their needs. If this is the case for you or someone you know, remember that there are many excellent swimming teachers who offer enjoyable programs for beginners of all ages. If you can't find one, make some inquiries about having one started at your local pool. A good teacher will show you effective techniques for keeping water out of your sensitive eyes, nose, and mouth.

For the reasons discussed above, injuries are uncommon among swimmers. They do occasionally occur, however, most often in the shoulders and the knee joints. Shoulder problems can be caused by the repeated abrasion of tendons when they rub over the bony structures of the shoulder joints, particularly when you swim butterfly and backstroke. If the self-tests in Chapter 3 indicate that you are inflexible in your shoulders, you should include shoulder presses (Chapter 5) before and after you start a swimming program. Breaststroke swimmers have fewer shoulder problems, but the breaststroke kick can be particularly stressful on the knees for some people. You can either modify your kick or avoid the breaststroke if you have a history of knee injuries.

Cycling

> *"Bicycling—the best thing Man has ever done."*—John Krausz & Vera von der Reis Krausz, *The Bicycle Book* (Dial Press, 1982).

You can include cycling in your program in any of the three categories of exercise. The two of us use a formal training approach to prepare for our annual cycling holiday, we use our bicycles in a functional way to run errands and commute, and we have cycled many thousands of fun miles in the United States and Europe during our vacations.

Two factors might affect your decision to use cycling in your exercise program. The first is the availability of safe roads in your neighborhood. Traffic-clogged roads and impatient drivers in some inner cities can be a potentially lethal combination for the defenseless cyclist. Potholes and broken glass also present hazards for even the most ardent rider on poorly maintained roads. The answer is of course bicycle paths; more and more communities are recognizing that providing bike paths can reduce congestion and pollution on our overcrowded roads.

The next important consideration is your willingness to purchase and maintain a bicycle in safe working condition. Strangely enough, it is generally the rule that the *less* you pay for a bicycle, the *less* maintenance will be required. Less expensive bikes are usually made from heavy steel, which will withstand a great deal of abuse. Apart from the occasional punctured tire, they usually need only a few drops of oil and a brake check every few months to keep them running. "Serious" cycling enthusiasts usually take a great deal of pride in the condition of their more sophisticated lightweight bikes.

Cyclists do occasionally suffer injuries. The most common ones are scrapes and bruises resulting from falls and collisions, but you can usually avoid these problems with common sense and defensive cycling behavior. A cycling helmet and clothing that covers knees and elbows are sound insurance against painful abrasions and more serious injuries.

There are also other types of injuries that are often avoidable. Most of these are the result of using a bicycle that does not fit the cyclist. If your seat is either too high or too low, you may find that cycling will be stressful on your knees. If your handlebars are too low, you may begin to feel discomfort in your neck and back, and you may also experience pain or numbness in your hands and wrists. More and more people who ride for exercise are beginning to realize that mountain bikes can provide a comfortable riding position, but road race and track cyclists need curved "dropped" handlebars that provide a more streamlined body position.

If you are not an experienced cyclist, seek the advice of someone from your local bicycle store or cycling club before you buy a bicycle. There is a great deal of camaraderie in the cycling world, and experienced riders are usually willing to help you choose a bike that is the right size and to help you adjust the seat and handlebars to fit your unique anatomy.

Competitive cyclists use cleats and toe clips to hold their feet firmly in place on their pedals. This allows them to use their leg muscles to turn the pedals as efficiently as possible. However, some cyclists become injured over a period of time as the result of locking their feet onto their pedals. Research in our laboratory has shown why this happens. Several members of the U.S. cycling team had routinely suffered from pain in the knees and feet for several years. A detailed clinical examination revealed that three of them were overpronators. Overpronation caused the cyclist's knee to be forced inward toward the bicycle frame during the powerful downward pushing phase of each foot. This motion interferes with the smooth gliding action of the kneecap and can eventually produce a painful condition known as chondromalacia patellae. All three cyclists were fitted with custom-made arch supports that reduced the tendency to overpronate, and they lost much of the discomfort they had been suffering. One of them went on to win a silver medal in the Olympic Games!

If you want to include cycling in your exercise program, you can learn a simple lesson from this research. Cleats and toe clips may help competitive cyclists perform better, but they are not essential for someone primarily interested in aerobic exercise. Cleats can severely restrict the natural motion of your feet, and unless you have them carefully adjusted they are best avoided by the noncompetitor. Toe clips can improve your cycling efficiency, but leave them slightly loose to allow your feet some freedom of movement. If you do not wear toe clips, wear shoes with soles that provide some traction to prevent your feet from sliding off your pedals.

If the tests in Chapter 3 indicate alignment problems with your legs and feet, seek some expert advice before you commit yourself to a cycling program. If you are already cycling, avoid excessive mileage when you feel obvious discomfort in your knees and feet.

In-Line Skating

This exciting and relatively new activity has enjoyed phenomenal popularity in recent years. According to the International In-Line Skating Association (IISA), there were 4.3 million people skating regularly in 1990. By the end of 1995 the number of regular participants had ballooned to 26 million.

Unfortunately, injuries do occur, but the good news is that most injuries are preventable. The majority of injuries are caused by falls and collisions, and according to the U.S. consumer product safety commission, two-thirds of all in-line skating injuries have been suffered by people who were not wearing protective gear. So be sure to wear complete protection for your head, wrists, elbows, and knees. If you suffer from low back pain avoid spending too long in a streamlined racing position with your trunk parallel with the ground. Skating fast may be exhilarating, but remember that the objective of aerobic exercise is to work at an appropriate intensity in order to gain optimum health benefits. Most people can attain an effective heart rate in a relatively comfortable position that does not involve excessive forward lean.

Try to locate a smooth, flat, traffic-free surface for your training program. In-line skating has already been banned in some locations where inconsiderate skaters were a menace to pedestrians, cyclists, and drivers. So use common sense and courtesy so that all of us can share and enjoy the many locations that are still available.

Finally, if you have not yet tried in-line skating, or if you are still a little unsure of yourself, we recommend that you join a class and take some lessons. Instructors certified by the IISA are trained to use effective teaching strategies that will help you learn to skate confidently and safely in a fairly short period of time. Not surprisingly, one of the first things that you will learn is how to stop! Even gifted athletes can avoid the frustrating process of trial and error learning under the direction of a qualified instructor. Remember, the sooner you can skate with confidence, the sooner you can start to feel the benefits of this exciting aerobic activity.

Cross-Country Skiing

This activity is not as popular in the United States as it is in northern Europe, but we have included it because it is extremely effective aerobic training. It is also remarkable because, although it is physiologically demanding, the mechanics of the activity tend to minimize injurious stresses on the musculoskeletal system. Cross-country skiing involves strenuous work both with the arms and the legs, and scientific testing has shown that some competitive crosscountry skiers have the highest level of aerobic fitness of any Olympic athletes. The obvious limitation for many of us is that cross-country skiing can be done only when and where snow-covered trails are available. Regular training is therefore out of the question for most people who live in warm climates. Skis, poles, and suitable shoes and clothing are also required. If you are fortunate enough to have all the necessary equipment and facilities available, you can use cross-country skiing as regularly scheduled formal exercise. Some people who live in remote areas are obliged to use it as functional transportation, and many aficionados of the sport use it as fun exercise in invigorating surroundings with family and friends.

Unlike running and aerobics, in cross-country skiing the feet are usually kept close to the ground so that the skis can slide across the surface, rather than collide with it. Fresh snow compresses and helps absorb more of the forces on the feet. The arms are used in a relatively natural fashion, as in walking and running. Therefore, injuries appear to be relatively uncommon. Of course, anyone who is inflexible will probably be injury-prone in any vigorous activity, but cross-country skiing may well be an ideal activity for many people who would find some other aerobic activities mechanically stressful.

Rowing and Paddling

Rowing, canoeing, and kyaking are lifetime sports that can be enjoyed by young and old alike. The mechanics of kyaking are such that disabilities of the legs do not prevent the exercise enthusiast from performing effectively. In fact, one of the truly gratifying aspects of this sport is that some of the world's most outstanding competitors have such disabilities. The great majority of people who take part in aquatic activities use them as fun exercise, but competitors must undergo a great deal of formal training to be successful. Of course, in wilderness areas these same activities can also provide a functional means of transportation. For safety reasons, swimming skills are highly recommended.

All three activities use many of the major muscles of the arms, shoulders, back, and abdomen. Rowing also uses the large muscles of the legs. None of them involves impacts to the feet. Water also tends to cushion forces that are exerted on the hands and arms by paddles and oars. As a result, the rate of injury in these activities is relatively low

The injuries that do occur in competitors often involve the wrist, forearm, and low back. The range of motion required in these activities has been described as more natural than swimming, thus rowers and paddlers seem to suffer fewer shoulder injuries than swimmers. If you have had problems with the tendons on the back of your wrists, or if you suffer from low back pain, you may be predisposed to further problems in these activities. It is believed that the repetitive twisting of the trunk during the powerful propulsive phase in kyaking and canoeing might be particularly stressful to someone who already suffers from low back pain. As a further precaution, you should spend some time improving the strength of your abdominals and shoulder muscles and improving your overall flexibility before taking up any of these activities.

Indoor Aerobic Exercise Devices

Various machines that simulate cycling, rowing, skiing, trampolining, and climbing are now available to the exercise enthusiast. These devices, together with the age-old favorite activity of rope-jumping, can be used indoors throughout the year. The comfort and security of your home or health club can help you maintain a regularly scheduled formal exercise program. Some exceptional people find that this is the best way for them to meet their exercise goals, but many others have found that the exclusive use of one of these training devices can be boring. Because of our preference for a combination formal-functional-fun exercise program, the two of us find that the most effective use of aerobic exercise devices is to provide some variety, especially when other facilities are not available due to bad weather and busy schedules. If these machines appeal to you, it is a good idea to mix and match activities. Rest those parts of your body that have been taking the most stress from your usual activities, and choose a variety of devices that provide different movements from the ones you do most frequently.

Any machine will tend to exert specific stresses on your body if you use it in your aerobic exercise program. You should take the precautions that were discussed for cycling when you use an exercise bike. You should consider the areas of the body that are most commonly injured in rowing if you use a rowing machine. Rope jumping and rebounders (or mini-tramps) involve repeated impacts to the feet, so you should review the sections in this chapter dealing with similar activities-running and dance exercise.

FIT TIPS

1. Regular aerobic activities can help reduce the risk of coronary disease.

2. Aerobic exercise is *any* physical activity that continuously uses the large muscles of your body for at least 12 minutes at an intensity that will produce cardiorespiratory benefits.

3. Select aerobic activities that you truly enjoy doing.

4. If possible, perform more than one aerobic activity during any one week. Cross-training (mixing and matching activities) helps relieve boredom and reduces the wear and tear on your body.

5. For health benefits, you should exercise aerobically at 50 to 75 percent of your heart rate reserve (see Chart 1) for 12 to 30 minutes, three to four times a week on alternate days.

6. Moderate levels of exercise will provide good aerobic benefits without exposing you to a high risk of injury.

7. Warm up and stretch before performing aerobic activity.

8. Cool down and stretch after each aerobic session.

9. If any physical activity causes you unusual pain or discomfort, *stop doing* the activity and consult a fitness expert or medical professional.

Chapter 9

HOW YOU CAN LOSE WEIGHT EFFECTIVELY

"I just need to lose 10 or 12 pounds and I will be real happy with this class."—College student, California

". . . there are a few things that I wish I could change: my upper arms or those too-short legs or that incipient double chin . . ."—Elizabeth Taylor, *Elizabeth Takes Off*

"I am so frustrated. I must have spent close to $1,000 over the last five years on memberships and I am 7 or 8 pounds heavier than when I started."—J. S., Las Vegas

"I am not overweight, I'm under-tall."—Garfield, a.k.a. Jim Davis, cartoonist

When we asked various people about their exercise goals, many of them told us they wanted to "lose some weight." In fact, this seems to be the number one goal of the majority of people who take part in exercise programs. That's why we have devoted an entire chapter to this concern.

Obesity

Generally speaking, when you are less physically active, you tend to eat and drink more, especially when your appetite is stimulated. These conditions also lead to a tendency to consume foods that are high in calories. In our society we have come to rely more and more on mechanized transportation and other devices that do physical work for us. This nation is also the world's most abundant producer of foods, and in an effort to keep up the demand for food, advertisers relentlessly bombard us with constant reminders of the joys of eating and drinking. Thus Americans are among the world's most inactive people, and we have the greatest temptation to eat and drink.

Of course, almost everyone recognizes that obesity is a serious health problem, so we are also deluged with more advertising for diet books and magazines, for "fat farms" and weight loss programs, and the greatest irony of all-for yet more food and drink. We are told that the answer to those sugary soft drinks and greasy foods is to buy an artificially-sweetened soft drink and "light snacks" from the very same people who sold us the stuff that caused the weight problem in the first place!

The national concern about obesity has also attracted the attention of some of the same entrepreneurs we talked about in Chapter 1. You have seen the ads for bizarre pills and potions that promise to "dissolve your fat while you eat everything you want," or to effortlessly "attack the fat molecules" in those places where you want to lose weight. There are contraptions that are supposed to literally "shock" your flabby muscles into shape and machines that will "vibrate" your bulges away. You can be sure that as long as there are people who are willing to spend money on weight loss, there will be at con artists eager to come up with new ways to help them spend it.

We have no such miracles to offer you. Neither does the rest of the legitimate scientific community. Even if a dubious product is "recommended by doctors," the manufacturers rarely tell us who those doctors are. For all we know it could be a doctor of divinity or a Ph.D. whose training was in archeology. Unless the first one has a direct line to a Higher Source or the second one has dug up something from a previous enlightened civilization, we can think of no reason that they should know any more than the average person about food chemistry. The best advice we have ever heard about diet is: If it sounds too good to be true, it probably is! The simple fact of the matter is that all the advice you have heard over and over again from sensible, well-qualified experts is true. The following paragraph summarizes almost everything worth knowing in all the diet books on all the shelves in your local bookstore:

There are two key factors to a good diet. The first is *moderation* and the second is *balance*. Don't eat more food than your body needs, and make sure the food you eat contains what your body

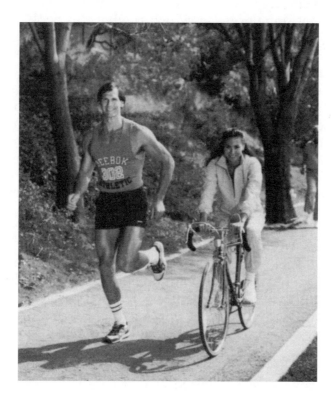

needs to stay healthy. On average, your daily intake should consist of at least 55 percent carbohydrates, mostly complex carbohydrates such as whole wheat bread, pasta, and vegetables. The fiber provided by complex carbohydrates is important to the health of your digestive system. When eating simple carbohydrates, choose fruits over cake and cookies. Your diet should also contain approximately 15 percent protein (meats, poultry, fish, eggs, legumes, and milk products), and 30 percent or less of your daily intake should consist of fats, preferably unsaturated fats that are found mostly in plant sources. Remember that many of the foods that we think of as protein (such as meats) are actually a combination of protein and fat. Eating too much saturated fat (found mainly in animal sources) increases your risk of heart disease. Eat a balanced variety of different foods and you generally won't need vitamin and mineral supplements. Use the salt shaker sparingly, and drink several pints of water every day. If you drink alcohol, do it in moderation. And of course, get some exercise, which is what this book is all about!

Physical Appearance

As with all other cultures throughout history, our beliefs, attitudes, and values are shaped by those around us. If you had been born a couple of hundred years ago in Hawaii, you probably would have preferred an appearance that would be considered greatly overweight by today's standards. Even more recently, the female stars of the silent screen are probably regarded as rather plump by most contemporary moviegoers.

For the past two or three decades, the preference throughout the Western world has been for "slim" women and "lean" men. This has probably evolved from a concern about the health risks of obesity and a high regard for athletic prowess. The fashion industry has reinforced these preferences by offering clothes that look best on extremely slender models. Leisure clothing lines are often designated as "sportswear," and athletes are recruited as models by the industry.

The endless parade of skinny models across our TV screens and magazine covers has convinced us that slim is beautiful. We have come to prefer the hollow-cheeked appearance of women who have minimal body fat. At the same time, our society has maintained the traditional conviction that men must be "manly," so they must have muscles. Many young women have indicated that they prefer men with small buttocks, long legs, and broad shoulders. Of course, one of the delights of adolescence has always been a good-humored amazement at the fashionable absurdities revealed in paintings and photographs of our ancestors. Have you stopped to consider the reaction of future generations to some of the anorexic-looking "beauties" and steroid-inflated hulks of the late 20th century?

For the time being, however, our society's attitudes and values include the convictions that slim and lean are in. Unfortunately, many people are confused about what is regarded as beautiful and what is healthy. The fact is that in some respects, contemporary preferences in appearance may be desirable from the point of view of our health and well-being. In other respects there is no doubt that our preferences may not be in our best interests.

The current preference for slim and lean bodies has raised national consciousness about weight control, and many people have come to recognize the importance of sensible diet and regular exercise. On the other hand, some people have trouble coping with the demands of meeting the expectations of either themselves or others around them as they strive to be the perfect "10." Medical experts have become alarmed at the number of women who have developed deep-seated psychological disturbances that manifest themselves in the form of eating disorders. In their efforts to cut down on calories, some unfortunate people keep themselves on the verge of starvation, depriving their bodies of the important substances that accompany those unwanted calories. Vitamin and mineral deficiencies pose serious health problems for the compulsive undereater.

What Can Exercise Do for Your Weight?

When people say they want to lose weight, they inevitably mean they want to lose fat. Fortunately, for most people a combination of exercise and diet can help control the amount of fat that

145

is stored in the body. Recent research has once more opened up the complex questions of individual differences in metabolic rates and the physiological properties of different kinds of fat cells, but the remainder of this chapter will be restricted to exercise and its apparent effects on "otherwise healthy" people.

Basically, your fat is an energy resource stored in different parts of your body. Most fat is stored in special cells that form adipose tissue, but there are additional supplies in your muscles and other locations. When you ingest more food than your body can use, whether it be protein, carbohydrate, or fat, the excess will be stored as fat. Understanding the ways your body uses energy supplies is the key to planning a weight control exercise program.

Under normal conditions, the body relies on two sources of fuel to produce energy—sugar (carbohydrates) and fat. During low to moderately intense exercise, a greater proportion of fat is burned compared to higher intensity exercise. In addition, your body burns a higher proportion of fat the longer the duration of your exercise session. This does not mean that any form of exercise will burn either fat or carbohydrate exclusively. The bottom line is that any fat that is unused after exercise remains as fat, and any carbohydrate that is unused will be converted into fat.

However, there are sound reasons for encouraging you to exercise at moderate intensities. The physiological demands and the mechanical pounding that your body sustains during high intensity exercise will probably limit the amount of time that you can spend exercising safely. Over time, longer sessions of moderate-intensity exercise can burn more calories (and hence unwanted fat) than shorter sessions of high-intensity exercise that may be painful. In other words, minute for minute, high-intensity exercise burns more calories than lower-intensity exercise, but in the long run you will probably be able to accumulate greater caloric expenditure with less discomfort, and fewer injuries, if you exercise conscientiously at moderate intensity.

A research study that we completed recently illustrates this point. Using a portable laboratory instrument that allows us to measure oxygen uptake (and hence, exercise intensity) we monitored a dozen young women walking and running on flat and hilly terrain. On the basis of our measurements, we compared the energy expenditure of running 30-minutes in hilly terrain, three days a week, with the expenditure of the same women walking on flat ground for one hour per day, five days a week. The results should tell you why we advocate low- to moderate-intensity exercise for a weight loss program.

The women in our study burned *twice as many calories* during 5 days of walking on flat ground (one hour per day) as they did running hills three days per week (half hour per day). Needless to say, your feet, knees, and shins will appreciate a gentle walking program, in spite of the fact that you will have to invest more time on a walking program than you would in a tough running program like the one we examined.

1. If your primary goal is to burn fat, low- to moderate-intensity exercise is the most effective and safest way to do it. There is no doubt that high-intensity training is essential for those whose goals include improvements in athletic performance, but frequent walking is a very effective way to help you shed those unwanted pounds. This is especially true for someone who is injury-prone or obese.

2. If your exercise goals include improvements in aerobic fitness and weight loss, you have three alternative ways to achieve your goals. The first alternative is most appropriate for someone who is extremely deconditioned and extremely overweight. The second is appropriate for someone who is deconditioned and overweight. The third is appropriate for someone who is in fairly good condition and not significantly overweight.

a. For the extremely deconditioned and markedly overweight individual, there is no doubt that the first priority is to shed some pounds. Weight loss reduces the mechanical stress on the joints and lessens the chance of injury. A low intensity program such as walking is appropriate, and the key to success is "little and often." That is, in the early stages, it is important to limit the mechanical stress, so short walks a couple of times a day are better than long fatiguing hikes. When the cumulative effects of the walking program begin to produce results, the intensity of the exercise can be cautiously increased. When moderate intensity exercise can be tolerated, the individual can progress to an aerobic exercise program.

b. Someone who is somewhat out of shape and a little over-weight may be unable to tolerate moderately-high-intensity exercise. However, this individual can still improve aerobic fitness and lose weight if exercise is kept at an appropriate intensity. Remember that aerobic fitness can be improved with sustained and frequent exercise at intensities between 50 and 85 percent heart rate reserve. It is impossible to calculate the "best" intensity for anyone, but within the range of 50 to 60 percent maximum heart rate reserve, the mechanical stress will be predictably less than at higher intensities. This range is appropriate for a deconditioned individual, and over time the duration of exercise sessions can be increased up to a maximum of as much as an hour. Over time the cumulative effects of exercise will help the individual to meet weight loss goals.

c. For someone who is in fairly good condition and not significantly overweight, the best way to reach the goals of improving aerobic fitness and weight loss is to incorporate two separate and highly effective training elements in a single exercise program. That is, one aspect of training will address aerobic fitness and the other will provide sustained "fat burning" activity. For example, 30 minutes of moderately-high-intensity aerobic exercise, (about 75% heart rate reserve) on Monday, Wednesday, and Friday will help meet the goal of improving aerobic fitness. Long-duration (in excess of an hour), low- to moderate-intensity exercise (at, say, 50–60% heart rate reserve) on the remaining days of the week would help to achieve long-term weight-loss goals.

We strongly believe that widespread misunderstandings about the relationship between weight loss and exercise were responsible for many of the injuries that occurred during the jogging boom. Many people who took up jogging were influenced by the widely quoted statement that it is necessary to train at an intensity between 60 and 80 percent heart rate reserve in order to get aerobic benefits. Unfortunately, aerobic benefits were automatically thought to include weight loss, so thousands of joggers whose primary goal was weight loss indiscriminately trained in the middle and upper parts of this range. In many cases they logged considerable mileage and eventually became injured. The sad thing is that many runners might have avoided injuries *and* also have been more successful in meeting their major goal of weight loss if they had understood the information we have just presented. For this reason we believe that the growing popularity of walking is a welcome sign. For many people, brisk walking can be sufficiently intense for weight loss, and it can be sustained long enough to effectively burn fat without an unacceptably high risk of injury.

Measuring Weight Loss

The most common way to measure weight loss is to step on a bathroom scale. Unfortunately, many people mistake weight loss for fat loss. Your scale can only measure total body weight—it can't discriminate between the separate weights of your fat, muscles, bones, or the contents of your digestive system. This means your scale can be extremely misleading when it comes to measuring fat loss. Let's look at a couple of examples that illustrate this point.

Sara wanted to surprise her husband by wearing her wedding dress on their silver wedding anniversary. But she had put on a few pounds, and it was now too tight. Sara began an aerobic dance program three times a week and also did regular weight training at her health club. After the first ten weeks, Sara was disappointed to see little change in her weight. In desperation, she decided to try on her wedding dress again anyway. Much to her surprise, the dress fit comfortably. Sara did not realize that while she had not lost weight, she had lost inches. As a result of her exercise program, she had lost fat weight but she had also gained some muscle weight. The scale was simply unable to show this difference.

Charlie was convinced he could lose fat by exercising in a suit made from rubberized fabric. After a vigorous game of racquetball with Peter, he weighed himself and found he had lost a couple of pounds. But the weight mysteriously reappeared a couple of hours later. The explanation is quite simple. Charlie's suit prevented his sweat from evaporating, and in an effort to keep itself cool, his body continued to produce more sweat. As a result, he lost a great deal of *water*. Within the next two hours Charlie drank a couple of pints of mineral water to quench his thirst, and his weight increased.

These examples are *not* meant to illustrate that vigorous exercise has no effect on body composition. In fact, quite the opposite is true. From available knowledge about the intensity of various activities, as well as a knowledge of your weight and how long you spend exercising, it is possible to estimate the number of calories burned during exercise. Let's look at an example, using the information provided in Appendix B. Suppose a 160-pound man plans to exercise aerobically for 30 minutes. If he chooses to run at a moderate pace About 7.5 minutes per mile), he will burn about 460 calories. The same amount of time spent swimming at a fast pace 150 yards a minute) will burn about 340 calories, aerobics will burn about 290 calories, and bicycling at a moderate pace 110 miles per hour) will burn about 200 calories. Walking at 5 miles per hour will burn about 260 calories.

We hope our examples have demonstrated the problems of using a bathroom scale to measure fat loss. The scale can be used as a general indication, but the mirror and your clothes are probably your most realistic guides. The next time someone tells you he or she has lost ten pounds in two weeks, try to remember what the person looked like two weeks before. Then try to imagine what ten pounds of fat would look like on your butcher's scale. In most cases you will be hard-pressed to reconcile one image with the other. If people who claim this kind of dramatic weight loss are obviously not that much thinner, or their clothes don't look a couple of sizes too large, they probably have not lost the amount of fat they think they have.

Sophisticated ways of measuring body fat have been developed. You can be weighed while you are suspended underwater, the thickness of folds of your skin can be measured with callipers, and the resistance of your body to the passage of a trickle of electrical current can be monitored. These tests require expertise and special equipment, and even experts disagree about the accuracy of each. For most of us, our mirrors and the fit of our clothes are sensible and reasonably good guides to the composition of our bodies.

If you have a SMART goal (specific, measurable, action-oriented, realistic, and timed) to improve your body composition, remember that each of us can be only what our genetics will let us be. We can control the total amount of fat stored in our bodies, but we can't selectively shift bits and pieces from one place to another. We can also tone up muscles, and that can give us a well-defined and firm appearance. We can improve flexibility and posture, and that will make us appear more poised and elegant. The best tools for measuring all these attributes of physical appearance are a mirror, your clothes, and a rational mind. The most important question you can ask yourself is, "Am I the best that I can be?"

FIT TIPS

1. The best way to lose weight is to combine a sensible diet with a safe exercise program.

2. Most people can benefit from reducing their intake of sugar and fat.

3. Fairly long sessions of moderate exercise are the best way to burn fat.

4. Burn extra calories by increasing your overall activity every day. Try walking instead of driving, climbing stairs instead of taking elevators and escalators.

5. Recreational activities such as leisurely bicycling, hiking, softball, or tennis are fun, effective ways to increase your overall activity.

6. Your mirror and the fit of your clothes are better indicators of fat loss than your bathroom scale.

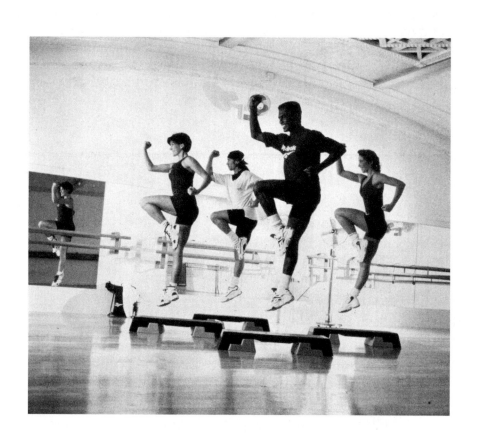

Chapter 10

PUTTING YOUR EXERCISE PROGRAM TOGETHER

"I've found all the right answers . . . but I've forgotten the questions"—bumper sticker

Now that you've read about the benefits and possible risks of exercise, you should be ready to design a program that's ideally suited to your own needs. As we have noted, exercise is like medicine. There are many different medicines available, but a wise physician will try to diagnose the specific cause of a patient's illness before prescribing the best medication for any kind of treatment. That same medicine might be ineffective or even harmful for someone suffering from an entirely different illness. Using the same approach, we have tried to show how it is possible for you to diagnose any shortcomings you may have before you prescribe an exercise program that will improve your health and fitness. Before we go any further, let's review each of the essential parts of a good program and see how you can use them to meet your unique exercise needs.

As a first step, it's time to check those exercise goals you wrote in Chapter 2. In light of the information we have covered so far, ask yourself, "Were they SMART goals (specific, measurable, action-oriented, realistic, and timed?" We've found that many people who try our approach discover their original exercise goals were too general. That is, you may not have been able to state *exactly* what you wanted to achieve. It is likely that if your goals were not specific, you would have no way of measuring them. After all, how can you measure something if you aren't exactly sure what it is you are trying to measure in the first place? If you begin with specific goals, you may find that some of the techniques we've discussed will now help you measure your progress. If your goals were not action-oriented, you would have trouble formulating a plan that would help you achieve them. When you have action plans, you should be able to estimate with some confidence how long it will take you to meet those goals. In other words, your goals can be timed. Just to be sure that your goals are SMART, let's review the overall picture of physical fitness.

By now it should be obvious to you that each of us may want to improve physical fitness for different reasons. In general, many people want to become fitter so they can improve their *performance*, while others are more interested in improving their *health*. *Performance-related goals* can be characterized by the Olympic motto, "Citius, altius, fortius" ("Further, higher, stronger"). In competitive sports, the object is to perform better than your opponents, but there are comparable goals for those who want to strive to compete against their own limitations. A growing number of men and women are trying to improve different aspects of their physical fitness so that they can realize their own Olympic dreams of overcoming physical and mental disabilities. Other people are driven to meet the challenges of mountains, deserts, and oceans "because they are there." The goal of going farther than you have gone before, reaching higher than you have dared to reach before, and being stronger than you have ever been before is indeed one of the most noble aspects of the human condition. In this regard we are all athletes of sorts.

Competitive athletes are often extremely good at setting SMART goals. Right now hundreds of determined youngsters have set a *specific* goal of winning a medal in the games of XXVII Olympiad in the year 2000. In each case the goal is very specific: a medal in swimming, gymnastics, skating, or whatever. Each goal is *measurable* with a stopwatch or a tape measure or by comparison with the criteria that have been set up for judging scores. These youngsters are relentlessly following carefully planned training schedules designed to bring them to the peak of their potential by the year 2000; thus their goals are *action-oriented* and *timed*.

Health-related goals are an investment in lifelong wellness. In recent years an increasingly large number of people have become extremely concerned about health-related fitness, and we predict that this trend will continue. A healthy body is better able to cope with the stresses and strains of our busy lives. Improvements in health can give us the vitality to meet the demands of home life, jobs, and leisure. In short, good health can improve the quality of our lives, and it can also prolong life so that we can continue to enjoy the health and happiness that each of us strives to find.

If you are one of the many exercise enthusiasts who is concerned about both your health and your performance, you can design an exercise program that will meet both goals. A well-designed exercise program can help raise the level of your *general fitness*. This can provide a solid foundation on which you can build other attributes necessary for success in your chosen performance activity. These additional attributes will improve the *specific fitness* for your chosen activity.

General Fitness

The most important components of general fitness are:

1. Musculoskeletal flexibility

2. Muscle strength

3. Aerobic fitness

People who have excessive body fat can be greatly restricted in their ability to improve the three components of fitness. Obesity can restrict the movement of the joints, it often leads to inactivity, which reduces strength and aerobic fitness, and the additional load on the musculoskeletal system can greatly increase the chance of injury during exercise. Finally, obesity involves a number of other serious health risks. Thus it is believed that for many people, a fourth important component in health-related fitness is body composition. As we discussed in Chapter 9, this component can be evaluated in terms of your relative proportions of bone, muscle, and fat. In particular, the ratio of body fat to lean body weight is important for health-related fitness.

A good general fitness program should incorporate stretching, strengthening, and aerobic exercise, and for people who are overweight, an intelligent weight loss program is essential. The results of the tests in Chapter 3 should help you design a safe and effective stretching and strengthening program, which will in turn help you improve or maintain good posture and efficient body mechanics when you perform everyday activities or any type of vigorous exercise. If you have been inactive for some time, you should gradually improve the resiliency of your musculoskeletal system with a pre-aerobic program (see Chapter 7) before you begin a strenuous program of aerobic exercise. A weight loss program can be incorporated into the pre-aerobic program if your exercise goals include an improvement in your body composition.

Stretching and strengthening should still be a regular part of your program *after* you have started aerobic exercise. The stretching and strengthening exercises we have presented in Chapters 5 and 6 are good general exercises that will benefit most people. When designing your exercise program, be sure to emphasize the exercises that were recommended on the basis of the results of your tests in Chapter 3. You will also want to include exercises that stretch the major muscles which will be used in the type of aerobic exercise you have selected.

Specific Fitness

The components of specific fitness vary from activity to activity. For example, gymnastics, diving, skiing, figure skating, combative sports, and dance require high levels of coordination and balance. Other activities, including ball games such as tennis, basketball, and volleyball, require coordination and balance, but they also require high levels of hand-eye coordination. Research has shown that these components tend to be task-specific. That is, if you develop the coordination and balance necessary to perform a somersault as part of a gymnastic routine, you will probably find it relatively easy to perform a similar somersault from a diving board. However, the coordination and balance you have to develop in gymnastics will probably *not* translate to the coordination and balance needed to shoot free throws more effectively when you play basketball. Quite simply, the best way to improve the task-specific components of fitness for any particular sports activity is to develop them by practicing the *precise skills* that are needed in *exactly the way they will be used in competition.*

Many other vigorous activities require the same components of fitness that are essential for general fitness, but they usually call for exceptional levels of one or more of these components. If you want to be successful as a weight lifter, you must become abnormally strong; if you want to be a good long-distance runner, you will have to spend a great deal of time improving your aerobic fitness. If you want to be a professional dancer, you may need extraordinary flexibility. You will need exceptional levels of more than one component in some activities. For example, successful gymnasts must be extremely flexible *and* very strong, and athletes who compete successfully in the heptathlon or decathlon must achieve extremely high levels of all components of physical fitness.

Of course, training methods for specific fitness for each and every activity are beyond the scope of this book. If your exercise goals are primarily related to performance, we would encourage you to take the advice of many outstanding teachers and coaches and add an additional goal of achieving a good level of *general fitness* before you subject your body to the rigors of training for high levels of *specific fitness.* There are many excellent references for training methods that can help you reach your specific fitness goals. Many of the national governing bodies that administer specific sports provide teaching and coaching programs, and they usually produce publications that can be an extremely valuable source of information when you plan your specific exercise program.

157

Where Have We Been Going Wrong?

After many years of teaching and research, and spending the last fifteen years carefully studying the phenomenon of exercise in this country, we have come to the conclusion that two overriding problems are associated with exercise at this time. The first is that many people expect too much too soon, and the second is that many people expect that exercise should be painful. Throughout this book we have tried to clarify these two issues.

The "Quick Fix" Approach to Exercise

Many of the people who try crash diets find that they just don't work for them. After months or even years of overeating and inactivity, some people decide it is time to lose weight, and they often decide they want to do it in a hurry. This rarely works, so they keep jumping onto the diet merry-go-round whenever another gimmick comes along. In the same way, many people who are generally inactive will suddenly try "to get in shape." In most cases they want to make significant improvements in a short period of time. All too often, people who want a quick fix either give up when they don't achieve the near impossible, or they persevere until they suffer pain or injuries that force them to quit. These folks jump onto the exercise merry-go-round whenever another exercise fad arrives on the scene.

Improvement in fitness is not something that happens overnight, but fortunately it is a realistic goal at any age. We would like to illustrate this with our favorite example. We mentioned Marilla in Chapter 7. Marilla Salisbury, who lives in San Diego, is in her mid-eighties. At the age of 70 she could not bend over to tie her shoes, and arthritis in her neck made it difficult for her to drive. Marilla was passing through our campus when she saw a group of older people taking part in the university Adult Fitness Program. Shortly afterward she became a regular participant in the program, but it took two years of conscientious stretching and strengthening and cautious increases in activity before she was ready for continuous aerobic exercise. At the age of 72 she began to compete as a runner. This remarkable woman now holds almost every world record in walking and running for her age group, she has competed on six continents, and she received an Honorary Presidential Sports and Fitness Award from President Reagan for serving as "an inspiration to all in demonstrating the true meaning of sports and fitness."

Marilla is a wonderful role model for many reasons. She started exercising a lot later than many of us, but she still made remarkable progress. Just think what you can accomplish in the rest of your life time. Marilla also did it the *right* way! She worked regularly on stretching and strengthening, she gradually built up the resiliency of her musculoskeletal system, and she avoided any sudden increases in the amount of exercise she was doing. Finally, she learned to love to exercise. She travels extensively and she continues to exercise wherever she goes.

If It Hurts, Don't Do It

If your exercise goals are primarily health-related, the title of this section should be the guiding principle throughout your exercise program. If something hurts, something is wrong! As we have noted, your body will feel discomfort when it responds to the physiological stress of exercise, but pain is your body's way of warning you that it is being abused. If a particular stretching or strengthening exercise causes you pain, then either your unique anatomy is incompatible with that body position or you are performing the exercise incorrectly. Find an alternative exercise or consult a fitness expert who can help determine if you are doing the exercise improperly or whether you're anatomically unsuited for that exercise. If you begin to feel pain in some part of your body during aerobic exercise, don't wait until it becomes a serious injury. Change your activity for a while or if you have made a sudden increase in your training, reduce the amount of exercise until your symptoms disappear. Mixing-and-matching activities can help to reduce the chance of a reoccurrence. It has been suggested that you should not wait longer than a couple of weeks before seeking medical advice if the pain does not disappear.

If your exercise goals are performance related, you must decide on the price you are prepared to pay for success. If you are prepared to suffer pain when you struggle to lift progressively heavier and heavier weights during your strength training program, you are not enduring the pain for the sake of your health. When your head is pounding, your muscles are burning and you are fighting for each agonizing breath of air during the last 100 meters of a 5K race, you are not enduring the pain for the sake of your health.

However, if your goals are performance related and you are prepared to tolerate pain if it will help you to succeed you should avoid the mistake of thinking that *all* of your exercise should be painful. It is extremely important that weight lifters and runners should be flexible and the guidelines for stretching are the same whether you are interested in health or performance. If it hurts, don't do it! For health's sake, the successful weight lifter should also do some aerobic exercise, but weight-lifting performance cannot be improved by suffering pain during participation in aerobic activities. Similarly, the long-distance runner does not stand to gain anything by suffering pain during strength training sessions. The best advice we can give you is, "Learn to listen to your body—it's the best teacher you will ever have!"

Sticking with Your Program

The best exercise program is a lifetime commitment to fitness and good health. A lifetime is a long time for most of us, so it is extremely important that you select an exercise program you can live with. If you choose unrealistic goals or indiscriminate exercises to achieve your goals, you will not be successful with your program. It won't be long before your exercise bike or set of weights are in your next garage sale. You should also choose a program you're comfortable with, a program you actually enjoy and look forward to. If you find that you become bored with swimming, give up swimming for a while, but don't quit exercising. There are so many different physical activities to choose from.

Earlier on we said that exercise is like medicine, in that it should be prescribed to meet your own unique goals. To take this analogy one step further, one of the reasons you might dislike medicine is that it can taste bad or have unpleasant side effects. Many people dislike exercise because they see exercise as medicine that does not feel good. Remember the advice of Mary Poppins "A spoonful of sugar helps the medicine go down." For many people, formal exercise is a chore, and they would rather be doing other important things or having fun. If you are not one of those people who thrives on regular formal exercise, we strongly recommend that you "sweeten" your program by putting an emphasis on functional and fun ways of staying active. The results of recent research indicate that you can effectively reduce your risk of having a heart attack if your exercise program includes moderately vigorous functional activities like gardening, housework,and climbing stairs, or recreational activities that involve walking. Every form of activity helps! As we've mentioned before, mixing and matching activities is less stressful on the musculoskeletal system and it relieves boredom. Variety is the spice of exercise!

What other strategies will help you stick to your program? You know yourself better than any other person. You must rely on your physical, mental, social, and spiritual needs and interests to determine the best exercise program for you. For example, are you a solitary or a sociable person? Solitary people prefer the pleasure of their own company, so they are most likely to exercise at home with a videotape than a sociable aerobic dancer, who would probably join a health club program. If you like to use exercise as a time to plan your day, reflect on things that are important to you, or even escape from the noise of others, you will probably prefer to exercise alone during some of your exercise sessions. If you find it easy to make yourself exercise regularly and go the distance, you are probably a solitary exerciser. But if you need that little extra push to get you going, you will probably function better exercising with others.

At the beginning of Chapter 1 we told you that 40 to 50 percent of the people who start exercise programs drop out within six months to one year. People who have SMART goals are much less likely to be exercise dropouts than people who are looking for a quick fix. We all have human failings, however, so it is wise to plan ahead and make sure that you will always be motivated to pursue your exercise goals.

One of the most exciting aspects of a successful exercise program is that it can provide its own motivation. One of Lorna's students recently wrote, "The thing that made this class so special was that I saw measurable changes in my fitness over the course of the semester." As you continually re-evaluate yourself with the tests in Chapter 3, you will be able to follow your progress. If you make discriminate choices of the activities you use to build up the resiliency of your musculoskeletal system, control your weight, or eventually improve your aerobic fitness, you will also find that they will feel good. After all, you will have chosen them because they are effective and enjoyable.

When we asked people who obviously enjoy their exercise programs what they do to "sweeten" the time they spend doing their favorite activities, they described some interesting ways they have used to keep their motivation high. One of the most common motivators, especially for music lovers, is listening to favorite tapes or compact discs on portable audio players. Other people enjoy listening to self-improvement audiotapes.

A number of busy professionals told us that they do some of their most creative work while they exercise. In the words of one of them, "After I sat in the office for almost a week wrestling with a design problem, I went for a run to clear my head. The solution came to me ike a bolt from the blue." Other people practice a foreign language, rehearse for interviews, review stress management procedures, or try to implement other personal growth practices. Several sections of this book were conceived during and after some of our early morning walks.

Many people have found that exercise becomes particularly enjoyable when it is part of their social life. We know of one interesting bunch who has weekly exercise get-togethers followed by a health food potluck. Changing the location of these social events from week to week and changing the activities from time to time keeps everyone's interest high. You can also combine exercise with some of your other interests. Some friends of ours who are enthusiastic gardeners vary the route of their daily walk to check the progress of plants and lawns around the neighborhood. Another friend always walks the eight miles round trip to the ball park when he goes to watch our local baseball team.

Some Final Thoughts

There is no doubt that you are likely to make a lifetime commitment to exercise if you understand *why* you need to exercise and *what* you have to do to make exercise safe, enjoyable, and effective. Historically, most human beings had to work hard to survive. Just two or three generations ago, most Americans had neither the time nor the need for formal exercise. Now we enjoy the sedentary comforts of modern civilization, and many people are not getting enough physical activity to keep their bodies healthy.

Modern science has presented us with some dubious short-term remedies. If your joints are sore because your unused muscles are becoming tighter and tighter, you can take pain-relieving pills. If your back aches because your stomach muscles are weak, you can sip a large martini in a hot tub. If your inactive body can't use food at the rate you consume it, you can turn to liposuction surgery to suck out your fat.

The shortcoming of all these remedies is that they will not treat the underlying *cause* of your problems. They simply treat the immediate consequences, and the problems become progressively worse unless they are resolved. In other words, these short-term solutions are just like borrowing money to get out of debt. You end up owing more interest! The health problems of many people can be avoided with regular exercise. The human body needs regular exercise, and without it it will continue to have health problems. The discoveries of modern science can keep us alive longer than at any other time in history, but many people will spend many of their added years suffering from the effects of inactivity. These are the compelling reasons there is such a pressing need for rational exercise. You now know what you can do about it. If this book has enlightened you about ways you can improve the quality and length of your life with a personalized program of enjoyable exercise, we will have achieved one of our most important professional goals. We wish you many years of happy, pain-free exercise and the healthy long life it can bring.

FIT TIPS

1. Set your exercise goals (Chapter 2).

2. Perform the tests in Chapter 3 and then design an exercise program to correct any deficiencies you find.

3. Design a personal stretching program (Chapter 5). Stretch daily to maintain good posture and reduce the risk of common musculoskeletal aches and pains.

4. Regardless of fitness level or the activities performed, almost everyone in our society should stretch shoulders, chest, lower back, front of thighs, back of thighs, front of hips, and calves.

5. Design a personal strength program (Chapter 6). Strengthen specific muscles one, two, or three times a week. Skip a day between strength training sessions.

6. Regardless of fitness level or the activities performed, most people in our society should regularly strengthen their abdominals and the upper back muscles to avoid aches and pains in the low back and neck.

7. Perform pre-aerobic activities (Chapter 7) for at least six to eight weeks if you have been inactive, recently injured, or are planning to start a new physical activity.

8. Select pre-aerobic activities that are fun, leisurely, and do not make you out of breath. Warm-up before engaging in pre-aerobic activities and progress cautiously, beginning with five to ten minutes of exercise and increasing five to ten minutes as your present exercise program starts to feel comfortable to you.

9. Perform aerobic activities (Chapter 8) three or four times a week, for 12 to 30 minutes at an intensity of 50 to 75 percent heart rate reserve (see Chart 1). Select activities that you enjoy and try to mix and match various activities as much as possible.

10. Find the combination of formal, functional, and fun exercise that works best for you.

11. Begin your aerobic activity by combining moderate levels of activity with more vigorous exercise. For example, if you choose to jog, use a combination of walking and running. When first starting your exercise program, walk a few minutes, then run a few minutes for a total of 10 to 15 minutes of activity. As you become more comfortable with the exercise, walk less and run more.

12. Progress cautiously. The rate at which you progress depends on your present aerobic fitness level. In the early stages of an aerobic fitness program, you should try to increase the length of your workouts by no more than a couple of minutes at a time whenever you feel you can work longer. As your fitness improves, you may be able to increase the length of workout by 5 to 10 minutes. Remember that 30 minutes of aerobic exercise is sufficient for most people whose goals are health-related.

13. If your primary goal is to lose fat, combine a sensible diet with an exercise program (Chapter 9). Longer-duration, lower-intensity activities will allow you to accumulate greater fat loss and minimize the risk of injury.

14. The fit of your clothes and a mirror are a better indicator of fat loss than is a weight scale.

15. Finally, *if it hurts, don't do it.* If you are in pain, your body is telling you something is wrong. Listen to your body and stop doing the activity. Seek the advice of a fitness expert or a medical professional.

Appendix A

TARGET HEART RATE RANGE FOR AEROBIC EXERCISE

For those of you whose heart rates and ages are not on the Target Heart Rate Chart in Chapter 8, use this easy formula to calculate your own target heart rate range using your age and resting heart rate range (RHR).

- 50% of heart rate reserve:
  220 – your age – RHR × 0.6 + RHR ÷ 6

- 75% of heart rate reserve:
  220 – your age – RHR × 0.75 + RHR ÷ 6

Let's take an example:

Sam is 22 years old with a resting heart rate of 45 beats per minute. This is how he calculates his target heart rate range:

1. Sam subtracts his age from 220 to get his estimated maximum heart rate: 220 – 22 = 198.
2. He then subtracts his resting heart rate from his maximum heart rate: 198 – 45 = 153.
3. Sam multiplies his answer in step 2 by 0.5: 153 × 0.5 = 91.8.
4. Next he adds his resting heart rate to his answer in step 3 to give him his one-minute exercise heart rate: 76.5 + 45 = 121.5 which he rounds up to 122 beats per minute.
5. Finally, Sam divides his answer by 6 to give him a ten-second exercise heart rate: 122 ÷ 6, which is approximately 20.
6. Sam then repeats step 3, multiplying 91.8 by 0.75 to give him the upper range of this training zone: 91.8 × 0.75 = 68.9. He completes steps 4 and 5 as follows: 68.9 + 45 = 113.9, which rounds up to 114; 114 ÷ 6 = 19.
7. Sam's target heart rate range is 19 to 23 for a ten-second count.

CALORIES BURNED FOR 30 CONTINUOUS MINUTES OF VARIOUS PHYSICAL ACTIVITIES

ACTIVITY	YOUR WEIGHT (lbs.)									
	80	100	120	140	160	180	200	220	240	260
AEROBICS	14	180	216	252	288	324	360	396	432	468
BICYCLING *moderate* (10 mph or 6 min/mile)	100	125	150	175	200	225	250	275	300	325
fast (13 mph or 4.6 min/mile)	160	200	240	280	320	360	400	440	480	520
CANOEING (2.5 mph)	56	70	84	98	112	126	140	154	168	182
(4 mph)	112	140	168	196	224	252	280	308	336	364
CROSS-COUNTRY SKIING	160	200	240	280	320	360	400	440	480	520
GOLF	72	90	108	126	144	162	180	198	216	234
HIKING *average pace* (3 mph or 10 min/mile) 20 lb. load	152	190	228	266	304	342	380	418	456	494
10 lb. load	136	170	204	238	272	306	340	374	408	442
no weight	128	160	192	224	256	288	320	352	384	416

ACTIVITY	YOUR WEIGHT (lbs.)									
	80	100	120	140	160	180	200	220	240	260
RACQUETBALL	152	190	228	266	304	342	380	418	456	494
RUNNING										
slow (6 mph or 10 min/mile)	172	215	258	301	344	387	430	473	516	559
moderate (8 mph or 7.5 min min/mile)	232	290	348	406	464	522	580	638	696	754
fast (10 mph or 6 min/mile)	288	360	432	504	576	648	720	792	864	936
SLIDE TRAINING										
basic slide	120	150	180	210	240	270	300	330	360	390
low profile	214	268	321	375	429	482	536	590	643	697
STAIR CLIMBING	176	220	264	308	352	396	440	484	528	572
STEP TRAINING										
4-inch step (simple choreography)	114	143	172	200	229	257	286	315	343	372
8-inch step (advanced choreography)	171	215	258	300	344	386	429	473	515	558
SWIMMING										
slow (25 yards per minute)	96	120	144	168	192	216	240	264	288	312
fast (50 yards per minute)	168	210	252	294	336	378	420	462	504	546
TENNIS										
moderate	112	140	168	196	224	252	280	308	336	364
vigorous	144	180	216	252	288	324	360	396	432	468
WALKING (5 mph or 12 min/mile)	128	160	192	224	256	288	320	352	384	416

EXERCISE GOALS

1. Your specific exercise goal or goals:

2. How will you measure these goals?

3. What's your action plan?
   (a) General action plan

   (b) Typical weekly action plan

4. Are you convinced this action plan is realistic? Why?

5. On what date will you achieve your goal or goals?

Appendix D

SAMPLE BEGINNER PROGRAM

Steve is a 35-year-old computer analyst who sits at a terminal most of the day and has not formally exercised since he played intramural basketball in college. Steve's exercise goals are to lose 10 pounds and to improve his aerobic fitness. He has decided to try jogging. Since Steve is deconditioned, he will need to begin with a pre-aerobic program and should exercise only 3 times a week on alternate days.

Activity	Time
Warm-up • walking in place while doing gentle arm circles	1 minute
Stretch • chest • shoulders • front of hips • low back • front of thighs • back of thighs • calves	4 minutes
Pre-aerobic • Week 1–2: Walk leisurely	10 minutes
• Week 2–4: Walk leisurely	15–20 minutes
• Week 5–6: Walk briskly	15–20 minutes

Activity	Time
Aerobic	
• Warm-up: walk	1–2 minutes
• Week 7: Walk 2 minutes/jog 2 minutes	10 minutes
• Week 8: Walk 1 minute/jog 3 minutes	12 minutes
• Week 9–10: Jog at 60% intensity	12 minutes
• Week 11–12: Jog at 60% intensity	15 minutes
• Week 13–14: Jog at 60% intensity	20 minutes
• Week 15–16: Jog at 60% intensity	25 minutes
• Week 16: Jog at 60% intensity	30 minutes
Strength	5 minutes
• upper back	
• abdominals	
• shins	
Stretch	5 minutes
• chest	
• shoulders	
• front of hips	
• lowback	
• front of thighs	
• back of thighs	
• calves	

SAMPLE INTERMEDIATE PROGRAM

Chuck is a 28-year-old construction worker who has been regularly jogging 3 miles 3 times a week for the past 6 months. Chuck's goals are to continue to improve his aerobic fitness. He has decided to challenge himself by jogging a little longer each day, but he also wants to add walking to his program on weekends for the pleasure of it.

Activity	Time
Warm-up • walking while doing gentle arm circles	1 minute
Stretch • chest • shoulders • front of hips • low back • front of thighs • back of thighs • calves	4 minutes
Aerobic • warm-up: walk • jog at 65%–75% intensity (M-W-F)	1–2 minutes 30 minutes
Recreational • walk leisurely (Sat or Sun)	30 minutes

Activity	Time
Strength • upper back • abdominals • shins	5 minutes
Stretch • chest • shoulders • front of hips • low back • front of thighs • back of thighs • calves	5 minutes

SAMPLE ADVANCED PROGRAM

Jessica is a 45-year-old executive in a major corporation. She has always been active and has been dancing regularly for the past 5 years. Jessica's exercise goals are to maintain her present body weight and physical fitness level. She likes to exercise formally Monday through Friday and recreationally on Saturday and Sunday.

Activity	Time
Warm-up • gentle arm and leg movements to music	1 minute
Stretch • chest • shoulders • front of hips • low back • front of thighs • back of thighs • calves	4 minutes
Aerobic • Warm-up • Aerobic dance 75% intensity (M-W-F) • Bicycle at 75% intensity (Tu-Th)	 1–2 minutes 30 minutes 30 minutes
Recreational • Hiking/biking leisurely (Sat-Sun)	 60 minutes

Activity	Time
Strength • upper back • abdominals • shins	5 minutes
Stretch • chest • shoulders • front of hips • low back • front of thighs • back of thighs • calves	5 minutes

Appendix G

EXERCISE DIARY

Exercise Goals:

Exercises and Physical Activities:
Flexibility   Strength   Pre-Aerobic/Aerobic

Target Heart Rate Zone _____ to _____

Date	Stretching Exercises	Aerobic Activity	Duration	EHR	RHR	Strengthening Exercises	Weight	Sets/ Reps

- EHR = exercise heart rate (10-second count)
- RHR = recovery heart rate (10-second count)
- REPS = repetitions

SAMPLE EXERCISE DIARY

Exercise Goals:

1. To become more flexible by doing stretching exercises everyday.
2. To tone up my body by doing strength exercises every day.
3. To lose weight by walking leisurely 2 days a week.
4. To improve my aerobic fitness by jogging 3 times a week.

Exercises and Physical Activities:

Flexibility	Strength	Pre-Aerobic/Aerobic
Elbow press	Arm lifts	Walking (Tu. Thurs)
Shoulder press #1	Curl ups	Jogging (M-W-F)
Standing back curl	Toe tapping	
Standing hip stretch		
Standing quadricep stretch		
Wall press		

Target Heart Rate Zone __22__ to __24__

Date	Stretching Exercises	Aerobic Activity	Duration	EHR	RHR	Strengthening Exercises	Weight	Sets/ Reps
10-5	All	Jogging	20 min.	23	20	Arm lifts	1 lb.	3/8
						Curl ups	Body	3/10
						Toe tapping	Body	3/8
10-6	All	Walking	40 min	—	—	—	—	—
10-7	All	Jogging	20 min	24	20	Arm lifts	1 lb.	3/8
						Curl ups	Body	3/12
						Toe tapping	Body	3/12

- EHR = exercise heart rate (10-second count)
- RHR = recovery heart rate (10-second count)
- REPS = repetitions